Peter B. Griggs was born in Mt. Kisco, New York on 10 September 1960. He graduated from Source Academy in New York City. He then graduated from SUNY at Albany with a B.A. in linguistics. He previously published a novel, called *No Pink Concept*. He has been a resident of New Jersey, since 1999.

I would like to dedicate *The Paisley Jubilee Story* to my brother, Henry L. Griggs III. He has always been very supportive of me.

Peter B. Griggs

THE PAISLEY JUBILEE STORY

AUSTIN MACAULEY PUBLISHERS™
LONDON • CAMBRIDGE • NEW YORK • SHARJAH

Ordering Information
Quantity sales: Special discounts are available on quantity purchases by corporations, associations, and others. For details, contact the publisher at the address below.

Publisher's Cataloguing-in-Publication data
Griggs, Peter B.
The Paisley Jubilee Story

ISBN 9781649799159 (Paperback)
ISBN 9781649799166 (ePub e-book)

Library of Congress Control Number: 2023923249

www.austinmacauley.com/us

First Published 2024
Austin Macauley Publishers LLC
40 Wall Street, 33rd Floor, Suite 3302
New York, NY 10005
USA

mail-usa@austinmacauley.com
+1 (646) 5125767

I would like to thank my dear friend, Bobby Hudson, who gave me suggestions on editing my novel.

I would also like to thank my friend, Keith Knox, for inspiring me to write this book.

Chapter 1

Three months after Paisley Jubilee had moved to New Jersey he moved into a boarding house in East Orange, New Jersey. He had discovered this place while looking up alternative places to live at a friend's home in Bloomfield, New Jersey. His friend Harry Harrigan told him that his living with him would only be temporary, because his lease prohibited him from having permanent roommates. It could have been possible that Harry simply did not want to jeopardize their ten-year-old friendship by familiarity breeding contempt.

The owner of the boarding house helped Paisley to move into a house in West Orange, New Jersey controlled by Easter Seals. Until moving to New Jersey, he had thought that Easter Seals was simply a religious organization. He never realized that they housed mentally ill people as well.

There he began receiving $210 a month in city welfare, until his social security disability claim came through. When he finally got his first SSD check for $600 a month, Paisley was transferred to a three-bedroom apartment also run by Easter Seals in Newark, New Jersey. It was near the Davenport Avenue stop on the Newark light rail system.

Paisley realized how lucky he was to be living where he was. The staff was friendly. The rent he was paying very low. This left him much more spending money than that of people in his old boarding house, where you were given a mere $85 per month for spending money.

Every morning Paisley would awaken at 6 am. He allowed himself an hour to shower, shave and get dressed before a van service would pick him and his roommate Jeffrey up. Every morning after he got up to the sound of his alarm, Paisley would awaken Jeffrey soon afterward.

While he was in the shower, Paisley often sang his favorite song from the 1960s. It was called *Bumble Bee* by The Searchers.

Jeffrey was a pleasant looking, light skinned black man. He had a moustache and was about five feet and nine inches tall. He and Paisley were the same age, having both been born in same year 1965. They liked similar music and board games, but they were different in other ways.

Jeffrey finished high school, but he did not attend college as Paisley had. However, Paisley never let his being better educated than others become an excuse to be an intellectual snob. Some of the most intelligent whom he ever met never went to college.

Paisley left his bedroom and opened Jeffrey's door. Jeffrey was covered up to his neck with his comforter.

"Jeffrey, it's time to get up."

"Okay. I know. Sometimes it's hard for me to leave my nice bed."

After Paisley took a brief shower, he dried off and wrapped his navy-blue towel around his waist. He checked on Jeffrey again. He asked him through the door which was ajar "Are you getting dressed?"

"Yes I am."

Paisley dressed himself in a 2 X T-shirt, underwear, socks, sweatpants, and very comfortable brown shoes. They were Rockport shoes. They were a Christmas present from his brother Argyle's family. Because Paisley was diabetic, his doctor always mentioned the need to wear comfortable shoes to avoid infections. Diabetics got sick more often and took longer to recuperate from any illness or injury.

Jeffrey usually needed more time to do things than Paisley did. A few minutes later Paisley returned to Jeffrey's bedroom.

"Did you take your medication yet?"

"I'm about to do that," answered Jeffrey.

While Jeffrey went to the kitchen to take his morning medications, Paisley heard a vehicle below. He looked out of the bay window in the living room and saw a gray van on North 6th Street. It was the van that always took Paisley and Jeffrey to their daily program. The mental health program was called Campbell Care.

"Gabby is here."

"I heard his horn, Paisley."

"We better be going now! You know how impatient he can be!"

"I know. Too many people are in a rush these days. Rush, rush, rush and they still get nowhere."

Paisley and Jeffrey went downstairs from their second-floor apartment and reached the little sidewalk outside of the house. Paisley opened the black wrought iron gate and held it for Jeffrey.

"Thanks, Paisley."

Paisley got into the pearly gray van first and sat on the big front seat behind the driver's seat. Jeffrey sat in the back seat that ran the length of the back of the van. He always did that for no particular reason.

With his thick Puerto Rican accent Gabby said, "Good morning, Mr. Siesta and Mr. Oops."

He called Paisley Mr. Siesta as an ongoing joke about Paisley supposedly taking a lot of naps every day. He called Jeffrey Mr. Oops because of a night club they drove past every day that had the incredibly idiotic name of "Oops here it its!" It was the title of a recent hip hop song, which was destined to be another one hit wonder.

"Good morning, Gabby," said Paisley.

"Today, Mr. Siesta, get me a cup of coffee and a donut at Dunkin Donuts," said Gabby, jokingly.

"Okay," said Paisley. "How was your weekend?"

"It was very good. Do we pick up Mr. Kenneth today?"

"Yes, because today is Monday."

Next to Paisley was a brown wooden clipboard. On the clipboard were transportation slips from the van company for which Gabby worked. It was called Reliable Van. Everyone who was a passenger transported by them had to fill out a form with their name, address, and signature on it. Gabby filled in the odometer readings. Then each passenger would have their counselor sign the form on the bottom line and return the form to Gabby at 3:15 pm. That was when their program called Campbell Care ended its day.

Paisley filled out his form and handed the clipboard to Jeffrey over the back of the seat.

"Thank you."

After Gabby gave him a twenty-dollar bill, Paisley went into Dunkin Donuts and bought Gabby an old-fashioned donut and a small coffee. He got himself a carton of orange juice and two toasted coconut donuts, one for himself and one for Jeffrey.

"Thank you, Mr. Siesta. Now we go to get Mary Holiday. You have to be careful of her," warned Gabby. "She put two men in jail."

"She did?"

"One day she tells the police that she was raped. A guy says he doesn't want her anymore so she says he raped her. It's total bullshit! Loca puta!"

Shortly thereafter they arrived at Mary Holiday's house in Nutley, New Jersey. She was wearing her usual pink leather coat and sitting on the stoop outside her home. She walked toward the van and got into the passenger seat, next to Gabby, where she always sat.

"Good morning, everyone!"

"You said 'everyone' instead of saying 'Good morning, Paisley' and 'Good morning, Jeffrey,'" said Gabby. "That saves time."

"I'm too sleepy to say it the other way," replied Mary.

Mary looked at Jeffrey and said, "That's a nice shirt you have on Jeffrey."

"Thank you."

Jeffrey was wearing an emerald-colored polo shirt with an ivory stripe across the middle. He had a plentitude of attractive polo shirts. Being enviably thin, he had no trouble finding medium sized shirts that fit him. He also was wearing a nice pair of chinos. Jeffrey dressed better than most of the men at their program. Paisley was still a bit chubbier than Jeffrey and had more trouble finding nice clothes.

Paisley handed the clipboard to Mary.

"Thank you, Paisley."

"This is my territory," said Gabby.

Gabby parked the van outside of a Krauser's convenience store. There were many other stores in the area with a similar name.

"Would you get me a coffee, Paisley?" asked Mary. "Here's a five-dollar bill for the coffee and for you to get something. Do you want anything Jeffrey?"

"Okay."

"Get Jeffrey a zebra cake too," said Mary to Paisley.

"Knock three times on the ceiling and save the last dance for me," sang Gabby.

"That's two different songs Gabby," said Mary.

"Who cares?"

After Paisley returned with the coffee and little cakes, Gabby drove to Kenneth's house. It was a plain two-story house on a quiet side street. There were a large maple tree and a cherry tree out front. Gabby beeped his horn thrice.

Kenneth emerged from the house, wearing a black shirt and black pants. He got into the van. He sat in the back seat on the left side next to Jeffrey.

"Yo, Paisley!" said Kenneth. "Good morning, everybody."

"Good morning Mr. Kenneth," said Gabby.

"Good morning, Senor Gabby."

"This is Kenneth's territory."

Kenneth usually had a shaved head and face. He had a dark complexion and beautiful white teeth. Paisley often wondered how someone who smoked cigarettes so much didn't have stained teeth.

"Would you like a candy Kenneth?" asked Mary.

"No, thank you. I don't have a sweet tooth."

As they drove through Nutley, Newark, and Montclair, Paisley noticed that there was a street named Fisher Street.

"I have an aunt whose last name is Fisher."

As they continued on their way, Kenneth made his own sarcastic comment in response to Paisley's comment.

"Hey, we're on Claremont Avenue. I used to have an aunt named Claremont Avenue."

They were going to pick up the only Asian woman at their program. Her name was Nancy Kwan. She lived in a pleasant looking boarding home. It was constructed of red brick with a small porch in the front. They usually had to wait for her about three minutes while a staff person gave Nancy her morning medications.

"Why don't they give Nancy her medications first? Every morning we have to wait for her," complained Mary.

"I know. I told Miss Smith at Campbell Care to call her home and tell them to have Nancy ready by 7:30. I have other people to pick up after you five Turkeys, every day," said Gabby, obviously amused with himself. "Why can't your program pick her up in one of their fat ass buses?"

"The bus drivers said that she lives too far away," said Mary. "They said I live too far too. It's all Tom's fault."

"Nancy, Kenneth, Jeffrey, and Alex all used to be on Tom's bus until he said we all live far away. That's such bull shit," fumed Paisley.

Nancy finally emerged from the side door in her boarding house. She opened the side door in the van and sat down in the middle seat behind Paisley, as she always would. Paisley handed her the clipboard which had her transportation sheet on it. She always signed the form as they drove away from her boarding house on their way to Campbell Care.

"Do you look fancy today, Nancy?" asked Gabby.

Nancy said nothing. After being discharged from a hospital called Overbrook in Cedar Grove, New Jersey, Nancy had become taciturn. She had also lost some weight even though she had already been thin. Her face now appeared sunken and shockingly older. Paisley also noticed that she had been wearing the same white dress with blue roses on if for three days now. Paisley was going to tell Cynthia the assistant director of Campbell Care about Nancy's appearance once they had arrived there.

"My boss David Stein said I can't get rid of Nancy because he makes too much money off of her. So, I'm stuck with her."

David Stein was the owner of Reliable Van Company for which Gabby worked. While he was receiving his monthly Social Security benefits, Gabby worked off the books, He gave the money to his reliable daughter Eva.

"I really don't see any problem with picking her up," said Kenneth. "We get to program long before they start serving us breakfast at 8:30."

"That's true. When Kenneth says 'Yes,' Paisley says 'No.'"

"No, Gabby, you're wrong. When Kenneth says 'Yes' Paisley says 'donuts,'" said Paisley, amusedly.

"I used to have an aunt named 'Donuts,'" said Kenneth.

"Paisley is mayor of donuts," said Gabby. "And Kenneth is chief of police of donuts."

"What about me?" asked Mary.

"You are queen of the zebra cakes," said Gabby. "One day we buy you a one-way ticket to Africa where the zebra cakes come from."

"You're crazy, Gabby!" said Mary.

"Do we pick up anyone else?" asked Gabby.

"No," replied Paisley. "Someone called me around 6:30 am and said that Frank is not coming to Campbell Care today."

"Good," said Mary. "Then we'll get to program earlier."

"You'll still get your free breakfast any way. What difference is five minutes here or ten minutes there?" said Gabby. "The food isn't going anywhere."

The van was approaching Main Street in Orange, New Jersey when Paisley counted the money he had. He had eleven dollars including the money from Mary. He had enough to get Mary's coffee, Jeffrey's zebra cake, and two bottles of his favorite soda which was diet cherry coke. He always consumed diet soda because he was a diabetic for many years now. The cherry flavor covered up the after taste of the diet soda.

The van crossed Main Street and entered the driveway which led directly to Campbell Care. On the left was a Wendy's restaurant. Across Main Street was the pharmacy where Paisley usually bought the sodas that he drank during the day. It was called Happy Pharmacy. They eased his dry mouth, a side effect of his Paxill.

"Deanna better not show up today," said Mary.

"Who is Deanna?" asked Gabby.

"She's a fat ugly bitch who called me a 'homo' last week," said Paisley.

"Next time you see her tell her 'Besame mi coolo.'"

"What does that mean?" asked Kenneth.

"It means 'Kiss my ass,'" said Gabby enthusiastically.

They arrived at the parking lot for Campbell Care. Mary got out first. Nancy got out next, followed by Paisley, Jeffrey and Kenneth. This was the way that they always mindlessly exited the van, almost like zombies.

"See you later, Gabby," said Mary.

"Adios amigos," responded Gabby.

Paisley walked down the driveway of Campbell Care while everyone else entered the building to go to the "all-purpose room." The staff normally referred to that room as the abbreviation "the APR." It was the largest room in the entire building. It was where the lunch was served, because it contained all of the sturdy lunch tables, arranged in neat rows.

Gabby tooted his horn as he passed Paisley and Paisley waved back. Paisley had never been acquainted with anyone like Gabby before this. Some of his mother's now-deceased snobbish friends would have found him to be low class and vulgar. They would have made fun of his heavy Puerto Rican accent too. Limiting their social contacts probably made their lives much more boring in the long run.

It took very little time to get to the Main Street Deli where Paisley got Mary's large coffee and Zebra cakes almost every morning. There was a large selection of sodas and pastries there as well, but Paisley usually chose the same things. Having made his purchases Paisley would then return to Campbell Care. The whole process of going to and from Main Street Deli only took about ten minutes at the most.

Paisley, finishing his tasks, entered Campbell Care. He passed through the small lobby. It was painted a lovely shade of lapis lazuli. The titles on the floor were a midnight blue. The receptionist's office was on the left and the psychiatrist's office, Dr. Patel's, was on the right. Both of their office doors had little windows in them to monitor whoever was coming and going from the building.

He went through double doors into the APR. The APR was painted a pale blue. There were several brown folding tables lined up throughout the APR. There were plain black metal chairs on the sides of the tables.

On the right side of the APR were five counselors' offices. There was ramp on the left side that led to the employee's bathroom, the kitchen, and rooms 1 and 2, where group therapy groups were held. Next to room one was the door to the administrator's office. Next to that door was the large receptionist's desk.

On the right of the APR was also a doorway leading to a hallway. This hallway took people to rooms 3 through 10. The floor was covered with blue and white linoleum tiles.

Paisley walked over to Mary, sitting at one of the lunch tables. He handed her the coffee and fifty cents change.

"Thank you, Paisley. I love you," said Mary.

"You're welcome," answered Paisley politely.

Paisley walked over to a table at the far end of the APR. It was next to the candy and soda vending machines. He sat down on one of the many black chairs between Jeffrey and Kenneth. He started to drink his 20-ounce bottle of diet cherry coke which he had bought at Main Street Deli.

"Could I have your book of word finds?" asked Kenneth. "And a pen?"

Paisley pulled it out of the Prado Museum tote bag that his friend Alec Wang had bought for him in Madrid, Spain. He always carried it with him. He had a pen, a small notebook, his group schedule, and an "I YNY" change purse for coins. He needed the coins to buy soda from the vending machines.

"Thank you."

As more buses arrived the APR began to fill up with the patients of Campbell Care. There were about one hundred people in all who attended Campbell Care. Most of them lined up to get their breakfast, which was always served at 8:30 am. Breakfast usually consisted of hot or cold cereals, a small container of milk, a small container of fruit juice and occasionally a piece of fresh fruit. The breakfast was always handed to them on a plastic tray.

Later in the day, lunch was divided between two different groups. The first group had lunch in the APR at noon to 12:30 pm. The second group ate lunch from 12:30 pm to 1 pm. Paisley was in the second group.

"Are you sure that you should always take favors from Mary?" asked Kenneth. "I have a feeling this party won't last forever."

"You worry too much," replied Paisley flippantly.

"I wonder about that, dude."

Chapter 2

Paisley was fairly popular at Campbell Care. Besides Kenneth and Jeffrey, he also socialized with other people like Lois, Tim and Jim. Several other people always said "hi" to Paisley when they passed him in the hallways on the way to lunch or one of the many therapy groups everyone had to attend at Campbell Care. He tried to not overextend himself, however.

Campbell Care unlike most programs in New Jersey had a workshop. Although the pay was below minimum wage, the income from the workshop provided many people with a few extra dollars above and beyond their "pin money" from the boarding homes. However, the boarding homes in Essex County were notorious for taking most of their naïve tenants' social security checks. For about 95% of your income, they gave you room and board.

The workshop itself was in a large room. It had been a mattress warehouse before Campbell Care took over the whole building. The room had fourteen large folding brown tables. Three were against the left side of the room. One was behind a couple of gray partitions against the right wall. The other ten were arranged in the center of the room. They were set up in a formation of a big rectangle, with spaces between the two end tables. The spaces were like aisles that enabled workers to walk around the tables.

The ceiling was about twenty feet high. The floor was painted gray with six different colored triangles in the middle of it. Three gray metal desks were placed near the gray partitions. The workshop manager's office was on the wall opposite from the three desks.

The workshop manager was a pleasant looking Puerto Rican man named Juan Martinez. Juan was twenty-eight years old with a goatee. He was unmarried and about five feet nine inches tall. He was slender and Paisley thought that he had a nice ass. He of course would never tell Juan that he admired him in his tight blue jeans. Juan might accuse Paisley of sexual harassment.

The work for the workshop was not meant to be well paid. It was meant to be a way of familiarizing patients who had never held a job with the experience of working. It also gave patients with no previous work experience the chance to get something to put on a resume. They could get help with a resume in the prevocational group.

All of the patients at Campbell Care did not work in the workshop. Many were like Lois who was unable to work due to physical disabilities. Some stopped working or never started working in the workshop because of the low pay. Those patients were considered too demanding.

Anyone who committed violations of the rules at Campbell Care was pulled out of the workshop temporarily as punishment. These violations included such misdeeds like smoking in one of the seven bathrooms, hitting another person, or cursing at one of the twelve counselors who worked at Campbell Care.

Paisley usually worked behind the partitions with Jim Everett. Jim was an attractive 49-year-old black man with a caramel complexion. He had a mellifluous baritone voice. He was six feet two inches tall. Paisley was infatuated with him.

After Paisley came out of the closet to him, Jim once said something about himself that was curiously erotic. "I have big feet and big hands, so Paisley you probably know what that means."

Paisley and Jim worked together doing flours. What they did exactly was that Jim would take brown paper bags and put three together to make three layers. He would weigh the bags filling them on top of a small scale with white spelt flour. When the bag had five pounds in it, he would give the bag of flour to Paisley. Paisley would seal the bag with packing tape from a plastic tape gun. He would tape a label onto the bag. When they had finished two bags, Jim would place them into an empty box, then seal and neatly label the box. One day, like so many others, Juan popped his head past the partition that separated Jim and Paisley from the other workers.

"I need you two to do twenty today," instructed Juan.

"Okay, will do," said Jim.

Paisley felt very comfortable working with Jim. Jim was always respectful of Paisley and had no problem about Paisley's sexual orientation. After being harassed off and on driving his forty-five years of living it was refreshing to find a sympathetic heterosexual person like Jim.

What Jim did not know was that Paisley had divulged to Kenneth that he was in love with Jim. But he would never tell Jim himself about his amorous feelings toward him. He was afraid that Jim would reject him like other heterosexual men had done before him. Kenneth thought that Paisley should tell Jim the truth, but Paisley disagreed with Kenneth. For the time being, Jim would never know what Paisley really felt for him. Meanwhile Paisley asked Jim questions about himself.

"Do you have any children?" asked Paisley as they made the flour bags.

"Yes, I have four. Three girls and one boy."

"Where do they live?"

"They live with their mother in New York."

"So, you're divorced? My family has had many of them."

"Yes, my wife divorced me while I was in the hospital," explained Jim. "I didn't know about it until I left the hospital."

"What hospital?"

"Greystone."

Greystone was a mental hospital in Newark, New Jersey. It had been there for many decades. It was a more permanent facility than the any of the ones to which Paisley had ever been committed. Paisley had never been hospitalized for more than two weeks.

"What was it like there, Jim? Really awful?"

"It was okay. I was in the main hospital part for a year. Then I was placed in the cottages for a while."

"The cottages?"

"They were like little houses. I had three roommates there. I lived in the cottages for about two years before I was discharged."

"Do you ever hear from your old roommates?"

"You know John Romaine? He was there too while I was there."

John Romaine also attended Campbell Care. He was a French-Canadian man who would sometimes stand outside smoking with Jim.

"Did your family ever visit you?"

"No they didn't."

They continued to process the flours while they talked. Paisley almost felt like a reporter interviewing the subject for a news article. Jim patiently answered Paisley's many questions.

"Do you ever hear from your children?" asked Paisley.

"No, not that much."

"That's terrible. I don't see the point in having children if they don't comfort you. You're such a nice gentleman. I don't see why they would treat you that way."

"It really doesn't bother me. It is what it is."

"I think that's very sad. Your family doesn't appreciate what a wonderful person you are, Jim."

"Thank you, Paisley. These things happen. No one ever said life would be what you expect it to be."

"That's true. Well, I am at least glad that you are out of that hospital and that you came to this program. Otherwise, we would never have met. I think my life would have been less pleasant if I had never met you."

"God brought us together for a reason I guess."

As Jim and Paisley worked on their flours, Paisley could hear people on the other side of the partition doing sugars. What that involved was taking whatever sugar substitute they were given, either Splenda, Equal or Sweet and Low, out of little trays. They placed the sugar packets on a sugar board which was a large piece of cardboard with twenty-five rectangles drawn on them. The workers would put on each of the rectangles a packet of sugar substitute.

When all twenty-five rectangles had a packet on them, that board was done. They would count how many boards they completed at the end of that period.

Every day at Campbell Care the day was split into separate periods, just like classes in a high school. Each period including lunch was either one hour or a half hour long. A buzzer was rung at the end of each period. The workshop period during which Paisley worked was only a half hour long.

Near the end of the work period Mrs. Black, an attractive middle-aged black lady, called out people's names. Mrs. Black would write down how many boards that they finished onto a slip of paper with each worker's name on them. She gave the slips of paper to Juan, who was her boss. Juan then gave them to the payroll office to calculate each person's paycheck.

"Cornell how many did you do?" asked Mrs. Black.

"I did ten, Mrs. Black."

"Lucille Trimble?"

"Twenty-five."

"Eric Jones."

"Twenty, Mrs. Black."

"Mr. Henderson?"

"I did fifteen."

Everyone called Mr. Henderson by his formal name out of respect for his age. At the age of ninety-three, he was like a de facto grandfather to everyone at Campbell Care. He was a very nice black man whom everyone liked.

"Deanna?"

"Twenty."

"Doris Peabody."

"Thirty-five, Mrs. Black."

"That's a lot to do! Tim Gaylord?"

"Fifteen, Mrs. Black. Did I do good?"

"Yes, you did," said Mrs. Black encouragingly.

Tim Gaylord liked Paisley so much that Paisley often wondered if he was in love with him. Because Tim was somewhat slow, Paisley wondered if Tim really understood what he was saying. Paisley however doubted that Tim was really gay.

Tim even kissed Paisley once on the cheek when he hugged Paisley. He often asked Paisley to hug him. Paisley could not get his arms all the way around Tim's chest, because he had a big belly.

"Mrs. Black you're a tank," said Tim. "You're really a tank."

"Thank you, Tim," she said. "Leon Bach?"

"Twenty-three."

"David Bolduc?"

"Fifteen."

Mrs. Black stopped right on time. The buzzer rang loudly throughout the building, because this period was over. Because few of the "consumers" (as Easter Seals and Campbell Care called them) wore watches, the buzzer kept track of the time for them.

"See you later, Paisley," said Tim with a broad smile on his face.

"You too, Tim."

Paisley emerged from behind the partitions. Then Paisley walked past Juan's little office in the workshop.

"Good work," said Juan through his open door. "You and Jim are two of my best workers."

"Thank you," said Paisley.

Tim Gaylord looked over at Paisley as he put on his tan jacket.

"I love you, Paisley."

"I love you too, Tim," responded Paisley cheerfully though lying.

"I think the world of you, Paisley."

"Thank you. Mr. Gaylord."

"Factored within, factored without." Tim laughed.

"Okay, Mr. Gaylord," said Paisley hurriedly.

Paisley really had no romantic interest in Tim, but he decided to humor him out of sympathy. He thought of Tim more like a nephew than a boyfriend.

Chapter 3

Almost everyone who attended Campbell Care took psychiatric medication. Paisley also took medications for medical reasons because he had diabetes, high cholesterol, and high blood pressure. He knew these medical conditions were hereditary because his mother and his maternal grandfather had the same afflictions.

The person who prescribed the psychiatric medications worked at Campbell Care, part time. His name was Dr. Rajiv Patel. He was a Hindu vegetarian from New Delhi, India. He was not very tall and had very short gray hair. He was slender, probably from eating very little food with animal fat in it. He spoke with an Indian accent. Dr. Patel had a pleasant personality. Everyone at Campbell Care liked him a lot.

Dr. Patel had a small office off of the little lobby in Campbell Care. Across from his office was another small office for the receptionist named Ramona, a friendly, efficient Italian American lady.

Once a month Paisley would see Dr. Patel to refill his medications. He sat in the little office painted a pleasant, pastel blue. In the little lobby, Paisley waited on a white plastic chair for this turn to see the doctor.

"Hi, Paisley," said Carlos. He was a twenty-five-year-old Peruvian with glossy black hair. "How are you?"

"I'm okay. I'm waiting to see Dr. Patel. I need refills."

"I need them too every month. But I'm not really sick. A girl put a spell on me."

"She did?"

"Yes, back in Peru. She was a witch and she made me loco a la cabeza."

"She did? What medications do you take, Carlos?"

"That's confidential."

"I'm sorry, you're right. I was being too nosy."

Dr. Patel opened his office door.

"Did you shave today, Paisley."

"Yes, I did Carlos. Did you too?"

Carlos caressed his own face.

"Yes. My face is smooth. Want to see?"

Carlos always wore white button-down shirts and black pants like a waiter in a New Jersey diner. He stood right next to Paisley. He ran his right hand across Carlos' left cheek.

"I like that, man. But I'm not a homosexual like you."

Carlos laughed and exited thru the front door to go outside.

"Who's next to see me?"

"I am, Dr. Patel."

Paisley entered Dr. Patel's office, closing the metal door behind him. There was a big desk where Dr. Patel sat. There were a couple of bookcases with charts in them, and another chair in which patients could sit. Sometimes a counselor would occupy that seat in case the doctor needed an update on someone's progress with his or her medications.

Next to his desk was a small window which opened into the medication room where the nurse worked. She could secretly hand him medications that way.

Paisley sat down and glanced at the round white clock on the wall behind the doctor's desk. It had the word 'Welbutrin' on its face. The clock and Dr. Patel's pens were probably free gifts from representatives of drug companies who stopped by Campbell Care occasionally. He knew they were not patients there because they usually were dressed nicely in business suits or dresses.

On the desk was a phone with big buttons, a Rolodex, and a big yellow notebook that had 'P. Jubilee' written on the binder. Dr. Patel opened up the notebook in front of him. It was Paisley's chart.

"I'm running low on my Ativan and Seroquel."

"Okay. Your pharmacy is still CVS?"

"No, I use the one across the street on Main Street now. It's called Happy Pharmacy."

"I'll call them right now," said Dr. Patel, cheerfully as he picked up the receiver.

There was short break while Dr. Patel looked up the pharmacy's phone number.

"Hello. This is Dr. Patel at Campbell Care. I need two refills for Paisley Jubilee. Yes, that's his real name."

Dr. Patel laughed. Paisley was used to that reaction to his peculiar name by now.

"I need one for Ativan and one for Seroquel. Make that three refills for each. Okay, thank you very much. Have a blessed day too."

He put down the receiver and wrote something in Paisley's chart.

"That's done."

"Thank you, Dr. Patel."

"How is your depression doing? Are you sleeping okay at night?"

"I'm pretty stable. The medications I'm on seem to be working really well. I don't have any more nightmares."

"Nightmares? What kind of nightmares?"

"I was having nightmares about being back in school. It's the final exam and I forgot to study for it."

"I see. That's not too bad. If you feel that things are getting worse, let me or your counselor know about it. Okay?"

"Yes, I will, Doctor."

"If there's nothing else, Paisley, you can go now if you like."

"Thank you."

"You're welcome."

Paisley left Dr. Patel's small office. He walked through the APR. He passed rooms 2, 3, 4, and 5. He went through the big room 6 and the even larger room 7, where the workshop was. He passed the men's and the women's bathrooms on the left, and three of the counselors' offices on the right. Room eleven was right after the last office on the left. That was where his home group was every morning.

At this time, however, a group called "medication education" was being held. Medications' education was the only group that every patient at Campbell Care was required to attend by the Medicaid representatives. Every few weeks, someone from Medicaid would visit Campbell Care to ensure that everything was running silky smooth, like Carlos' face.

This group was always run by Holly the staff nurse at Campbell Care. She was a nice white woman with wavy gray hair. Her pretty blues eyes flashed behind her conservative eyeglasses. She had worked before in Greystone for many years. Therefore, she was used to the eccentricities of the emotionally impaired, in both English and Spanish.

It was near the end of the group. Paisley sat down in one of black metal chairs lining the walls of room 11. About ten other patients were already there, seated in a large circle. As usual somebody was snoring, which Holly seemed to ignore.

Holly had a persimmon-colored notebook on her lap. Some manila folders with brochures about different medications in them were lying on the chair next to her. She stopped talking while Paisley took a seat.

"I'm glad you could join us Paisley," said Holly. "How are you?"

"Okay," said Paisley. "I just saw the doctor. That's why I'm a little late."

"Today I am going to talk about Ativan whose generic name is Lorzepam. Does anybody take Ativan?"

A few of the people who were actually awake and not daydreaming raised their hands.

"Lorazepam is used to treat anxiety. It may also be used for seizures, alcoholic withdrawal, prevention of nausea due to chemotherapy, tension headache and insomnia."

"My generation, the love generation is going out," said Kevin, a 60-year-old light skinned man. "If you look at it from that view, it's totally normal."

"Thank you, Kevin," said Holly politely. "Can anyone tell me what drug I'm talking about?"

"Closeral," said Lois. "Excedrin, qualudes, angel dust?"

Lois was a skinny middle-aged Jewish lady. She often talked in word salads. Her odd speech pattern often annoyed people at the program. Holly merely treated her with well-practiced respect.

"No Lois," said Holly. "Kevin, can you tell me what drug we're talking about?"

"I can't keep this all in me," said Kevin.

"Roberta?"

Roberta just shrugged her shoulders.

"Ativan," said Paisley.

"Paisley seems to be the only person here who is actually listening to me," snapped Holly. "Maybe I should get some milk and cookies."

"I'm paying attention," said Mary, the lady who also rode on Gabby's van. "I am not like these other slobs. They're so weird and pathetic."

"Now for the side effects. Ativan can cause drowsiness, dizziness, lack of coordination, grogginess, headache, nausea, dry mouth, blurred vision."

"That's a lot of side effects," said Jim.

Relieving his own dry mouth, Paisley sipped from a 20-ounce bottle of diet cherry Coke. It was his favorite soda. He often bought a bottle of it at Happy Pharmacy during the ten-minute breaks between groups.

"I know," said Mary. "I sometimes think the side effects are worse than the illness."

"Ativan is not recommended for use during pregnancy. This drug is excreted into breast milk. Consult your doctor before bread-feeding," cautioned Holly.

"The milky way," said Kevin.

"What do you do if you miss a dose?" asked Holly.

"Call your doctor. Call 9-1-1," said Roberta, giggling.

Roberta ran her fingers through her short, curly black hair. She often rocked back and forth in her seat. Dr. Patel said it was probably a symptom of her schizoaffective disorder.

"No, if you miss a dose, take it as soon as possible. But if it is near the time for the next dose, skip the missed dose and resume your usual schedule. Do not double up the dose," explained Holly. "What are the side effects of Ativan?"

"Is there anything they can do about atrophy?" asked Kevin.

"No, Kevin. We are talking about the side effects of Ativan."

"Drowsiness, dizziness," said Lois. "Tunnel vision? I mean blurred vision."

"Very good, Lois," chimed in Holly. "You're paying attention today."

"Headache, dry mouth," said Paisley.

"What else does it cause?" asked Holly.

"How often do you have your lithium level checked?" asked Kevin.

"When did you last have it checked, Kevin?" asked Holly.

"Six or seven months ago," answered Kevin.

"It causes headaches and dizziness," said Mary. "See I really am listening to you, Nurse Holly."

"Thank you, dear. That is correct," said Holly. "So stand up slowly when you get out of bed in the morning."

"I do everything slowly now," said Lois. "I can't help it. I wish that I was younger."

"We know that already," sneered Mary.

"I'm slow as molasses sometimes," added Lois.

"I used to like molasses cookies," said Kevin.

"My favorites are chocolate chip cookies," said Roberta.

"Before the bell rings, I need to know if everybody signed in," said Holly.

She picked up her notebook and manilla envelopes carefully.

"Yes," answered Paisley. "I think so."

At the very beginning of each period during the day at Campbell Care, everyone was required to sign an attendance sheet. It was placed on a clipboard and passed around the room. The signing of the sheet proved that anyone who was assigned to a group actually participated in that particular group. It was one of the many rules imposed on mental health programs by the people at Medicaid.

After the buzzer rang everyone left the room. During their many ten-minute breaks a lot of people would go outside to smoke a cigarette. This was true whether it was cold, or hot, even when it was snowing. Some people like Lois seemed to need their cigarettes even more than food.

Paisley did not smoke cigarettes, while Jim, Tim, and Kenneth usually did. Instead of nicotine, his favorite vice was caffeinated soda from Happy Pharmacy. Fortunately, the caffeine did not affect his diabetes or his blood pressure. Sometimes Paisley would drink decaf iced coffee instead.

He hoped that someday they would all quit smoking. Paisley's parents had always warned his two older brothers and him about the pitfalls of smoking both cigarettes and marijuana.

Chapter 4

Campbell Care had a wide array of different therapy groups. They were supposed to be geared toward people with different psychological diagnoses and intellectual ability. For example, the lower functioning people needed groups about basic hygiene. Patients who had both mental illness and chemical dependency had twelve step groups. This was the case for all of the similar mental health facilities in Essex County in New Jersey. The only difference was that Campbell Care was privately run, while other programs were run by the state of New Jersey.

Most of the patients at the mental health programs were unaware of the differences between privately and publicly funded programs. The privately run ones received money depending upon how many people attended them each day of the week. The state-run ones received funding even if some patients only went there one or two days a week. Therefore, most of the patients at Campbell Care were required to attend three to five days a week. Paisley found three days a week to be somewhat tiresome.

There were likewise prevocational groups to help with finding a job for those who were ready to graduate from the program. There was a women's group and a men's group to deal with issues that are specific to gender. There were groups dealing with depression, anxiety, and anger management.

Paisley was diagnosed as having major depression and an anxiety problem. Most of the patients at Campbell Care were diagnosed as paranoid schizophrenics. Because Paisley's ex-lover named Boris had been a paranoid schizophrenic, he was already familiar with some of their symptoms.

Paisley was scheduled by his counselor named Eddy Aiken for groups that were helpful for his type of mental illness. The only therapy group that there would never be at any programs was one dealing with being a homosexual. Except for Paisley himself, most gay men and lesbians were reluctant to come out of the closet at their programs. It was hard enough dealing with mental illness by itself, let alone both mental illness and homosexuality at the same time.

Paisley walked into room 8 and sat down in one of the black chairs. They had no arms on them. That may have been intentional on the part of the owners of Campbell Care. Chairs with arms on them were more comfortable, and more likely for people nap in them. The American Medical Association probably frowned on people sleeping in places where they were supposed to be helped with their problems.

He was usually the first one to come to every group. He looked at the white round clock mounted on the wall. It was just like the ones in all of the group rooms, and he realized he was five minutes early. He took a sip of his soda and waited.

About ten other people came into room 8. The group which was going to take place was called "dealing with emotions." The counselor who was assigned to run this particular group was named Edward Aiken, but everyone called him "Eddy." He was a thirty-five-year-old man who was both black and Korean. He had a mocha-colored skin tone and Asian eyes. He was very exotic looking.

"How is everybody?" asked Eddy.

"So far so good," said Lois.

Lois often interrupted discussions with irrelevant subjects. She would frequently sit next to Paisley in groups, as she did this time. She always liked him for no discernible reason. That was one of her peculiarities.

"Are there any issues that anyone wants to talk about?" asked Eddy.

"How about jealousy?" asked Paisley.

"What is jealousy in your mind," said Eddy.

"I don't get jealous," said Kevin.

"It's like when someone buys someone else a gift and not you," said Violet, a pretty 22-year-old white girl with hair dyed blonde.

"Lord," said Lois. "Doesn't food connect with emotion? I read about synthetic food. Have you, Eddy?"

"No, I've never heard of synthetic food," said Eddy. "What does that have to do with jealousy, Lois?"

"You could be jealous of someone having more food than you," answered Lois. "Like when you're really hungry."

"You could be jealous of anybody for anything," said Mark. "It's like when you're in AA or NA and someone says he's been clean and sober for twenty years. You think 'Why can't I be like that too?'"

Mark was a forty-year-old native of Turkey. He had wavy brown hair and brown eyes. Having been a United States resident for 25 years, he had lost any obvious foreign accent that he may have had previously. However, he still said sexist things that he said men in Turkey thought.

"You have to understand the black woman," said Kevin. "She might commit suicide."

"It can happen when a relationship goes bad," said Violet. "Sometimes love goes wrong. Then nothing goes right."

"I had a bisexual lover named Boris," commented Paisley. "He was sometimes jealous of both my male and female friends even though I am not bisexual and not sexually involved with females."

"How did you meet your lover? In a gay bar?" asked Mark. "They don't have gay bars in Turkey."

"I met him though a dating service. It had a directory of personals. The last month of the ad appearing he responded to it. We wrote to each other for three months before Boris and I actually met on Easter Sunday of 1981."

"Did you say you have a boyfriend?" ask Lois.

"No, I don't anymore," said Paisley "Although there is someone at Campbell Care whom I have a crush on. Do you have boyfriend, Lois?"

"No, I'm single," said Lois. "I don't want to get AIDS, syphilis, hepatitis, or herpes."

"What is the difference between herpes and true love?" asked Mark. "Herpes lasts forever."

Violet and Mark laughed. Lois looked very confused.

"I'm not jealous of anyone at Campbell Care," said Violet. "I'm sexy and I know it."

"Jealousy is terrible," said Mark. "Jealousy can make you lose your mind and lose your health."

"But don't you think dealing with emotions involves food?" asked Lois. "You can have feelings about food, can't you? Like at a birthday party."

"Don't make a big deal about it," said Mark. "I wanted what he had, and he is successful."

"I see those guys in music videos," said Carlos. "They get all those beautiful girls. I'm jealous of them."

"That's just acting," said Paisley. "Those women could be all lesbians in real life."

Everyone laughed, except for Mark. He was still a little bit homophobic.

"Only you would say something like that," said Eddy.

"Admiration is the opposite of jealousy," said Kevin.

"More power to you," said Alex.

"What if someone won the lottery?" asked Paisley. "Would that make their friends jealous of them? Or would they be happy about their friend's good luck?"

"If the other friend gets wealth," explained Mark. "You'll still be his friend. That won't change anything if you're real friends."

"It is unhealthy being jealous," said Alex. "It only hurts the dummy who's feeling jealous not the other person."

"Be happy for someone," said Violet. "If they're doing good, I'm never jealous."

Even though her name was Violet, she never wore anything which was a shade of purple. The most colorful thing about her was a streak of pink in her artificially blonde hair.

"Is there any difference between jealousy and envy?" asked Eddy.

"Yes, there is," replied Kenneth. "There is resentment with jealousy. There is no resentment connected with envy."

"How do you think so?" asked Eddy.

"Envy is just a feeling of wanting something. That someone else had," explained Kenneth. "Jealousy is wanting stuff something some else has and feeling bad about it, that they have it."

"I don't know if that is true," countered Paisley, taking a sip of the soda which was his trademark. "I thought that envy was for things. Somebody has a nice car, or a bigger house and you want what they have. It's the old 'keeping up with the Joneses' stuff. And jealousy is for people like my ex-lover who was jealous of some of my friends thinking that I was sleeping with them."

"I understand what you're saying," said Kenneth. "But that's not exactly what I meant. Envy is less painful than jealousy."

"I think it depends upon what you're envying," said Alex. "Like wishing that you had Jesse's girl."

"How can I find a woman like that?" sang Mark.

Everyone in the room fell silent for about five minutes or so. That included Lois who sometimes talked a lot.

"Holidays," said Lois. "You can envy people who have more holidays. Holidays have food. That's an emotion."

"Oh, shut up Lois," said Alex. "You always talk crazy. That's why you have no boyfriend."

"Alex, please don't talk to Lois like that," snapped Eddy. "Respect your elders."

"That's really rude," admonished Paisley. "Lois doesn't mean any harm even if she goes off topic."

"She always goes off topic," said Mary angrily. "I'm so sick of her. I wish that they would transfer her to another program."

"Do unto others as you would have them do unto you," said Mark.

"Whatever," said Alex. "Is that another quote from the Bible?"

"Did everyone sign the attendance sheet?" asked Eddy.

"Yes, we did," answered Paisley.

Just then the buzzer rang, announcing that this period was over. Mark left the room quickly to get in line for a cup of coffee and snack in the APR. Lois who walked more slowly than everyone else was the last person to leave the room.

"See you later Lois."

"Okay, Paisley."

While almost everyone else went to the APR or outside the building to smoke a cigarette, Paisley went to the Happy Pharmacy.

He passed though the double doors in room 6 and onto the driveway that led from Campbell Care to Main Street.

"Hi, Paisley," said Jim.

"Hi, Jim."

"I like you."

"I like you, too."

Jim was as often one of people who hung around outside smoking. Paisley wondered how anyone could afford cigarettes on the meager amounts of money everyone received. They cost about seven dollars a pack, and the price kept on rising over the years.

Paisley's money situation was better than Jim's or that of many people who were patients at Campbell Care. Instead of paying about 90% or more of his income to rent, like those people who lived in boarding homes, Paisley paid less than half of his income to rent.

The boarding home residents only received about $85 worth for their monthly expenses. After paying his rent, Paisley had $412 for monthly expenses. $85 was not enough money to support a pack-a-day habit. It seemed cruel to him that the cigarette companies had such a hold on these smokers' small disposable incomes.

Throughout his whole life, Paisley often wished that all of the smokers would simply quit smoking. They all said, including his now deceased mother, that quitting smoking was difficult. Yet if someone who had been such a heavy smoker as Lois could quit smoking, why couldn't Kenneth or Jim also quit?

Paisley thought of this as he crossed Main Street to Happy Pharmacy. It was nice and warm in Happy Pharmacy. He walked to the left side of the store past the magazine racks and sugary candy. He opened the glass door on the refrigerator and removed a 20-ounce bottle of diet cherry Coke. He went to the cash register on the opposite side of the store where the owner Nelson was. Nelson was from Haiti and spoke French and English.

"Hi, Paisley. How is program?"

"Hi, Nelson. It's just business as usual."

"That'll be $1.25."

Paisley handed two dollars to him and received three quarters.

"Okay, Nelson. See you later' Mon ami,"

Paisley placed the soda in his Prado Museum tote bag and returned to Campbell Care. Paisley noticed that Jim was still outside. He was standing where he usually stood, a short distance away from everyone else.

Campbell Care was composed not just one but two buildings. They were attached by a breezeway that crossed over the driveway to the smaller building, which Juan used as a warehouse for the flour and sugars that patients used in the workshop. When it rained or snowed, smokers stood under the structure nearest to the double doors. Jim stood across the driveway at the smaller building.

"Hi, Jim."

"Hi, Paisley."

"That group we had about jealousy was very interesting, wasn't it?"

"Yes, it was. But I don't feel jealousy that much myself. Most Buddhists don't."

"Will we be doing flours in workshop Jim?"

"Yes. Juan told me so."

"Okay. Jim, do you ever think of moving back to South Carolina?"

"Yes, sometimes I do, whenever I miss my mother."

"How long have you been a Buddhist?"

"About ten years. We can go to the Buddhist temple sometimes if you want. It doesn't cost anything."

"I supposed so, Jim."

"Why don't you think about it?"

Jim took a drag on his cigarette. He exhaled a plume of smoke.

"Are you Jewish, Paisley?"

"No, I'm not. But my brother's wife is."

"Oh, I see. That's okay. I'm a Buddhist."

Chapter 5

There was one group on Paisley's weekly schedule which could be very dull or very interesting. It was called "reducing anxiety." Its main purpose was to get patients to talk about things that made them feel uncomfortable. Then hopefully a solution to the problem could be found. It could however take many periods to solve more complex issues.

Paisley entered room 11, which was one of the largest of group rooms at Campbell Care. As he walked to a seat, Paisley noticed that he was not the first person to get there. Lois and Jim were already present. Paisley sat next to Jim as he often did in any groups where both of them were. Being next to Jim made him feel very pleasant and secure.

"Hi, Jim."

"Hi, Paisley," said Jim.

"Did I ever tell you that I love flowers?" asked Lois.

"Most of the women I know like flowers," said Paisley.

The counselor Jackie Jefferson entered the room and sat down. She was carrying a primrose-colored notebook. Like most of the counselors at Campbell Care, Jackie was in her mid-twenties. She had recently received her Bachelor's degree in social work from Rutgers University in New Jersey. She was thin and had blonde hair. She liked to wear pale colors. This day she was wearing a denim skirt and a blouse the color of key lime pie.

"How is everyone?" asked Jackie in a pleasant voice.

"I mentioned daisies and gladiolas," said Lois.

"That's a good idea," said Jackie. "Why don't we go around the room and share with everyone what our favorite flowers are."

"Gladiolas," said Lois.

"Roses, red roses," said Mary.

"Roses," said Carlos. "Red Peruvian roses. My mom likes them too."

"Easter Lilies," said Deanna. "Even if they're at a funeral."

Deanna was a large light skinned woman whom most people disliked. She was in the habit of hurting other people's feelings. Everyone thought that she was a lesbian, even though she denied it.

"Sunflowers," said Roberta. "They really do follow the sun."

"Roses," said Jim. "Maybe that sounds boring."

"Daffodils," said Paisley.

"What color are daffodils?" asked Roberta.

"They're bright yellow," answered Paisley.

"Roses," said Robin. "Everyone adores roses."

"Hibiscus," said Lucille.

"Red roses," said Mark.

"Roses," said Kevin.

"Tulips," said Kenneth.

"And my favorite flower is definitely roses," said Jackie. "That seems to be almost everyone's favorite. That may not sound so original. But I don't care about that too much really."

"I also remember gardenias and tiger lilies," said Lois. "And when I was growing up boys used to sometimes give their dates an orchid for a corsage."

"What is a corsage?" asked Roberta.

"It's a flower that a boy would give to his girlfriend to pin onto her dress," said Paisley. "That was back in the day."

The conversation ended for a moment or two. Jackie looked around the room, probably to see if anyone was falling asleep.

"Is anyone feeling anxious?" asked Jackie. "That's what we were really supposed to talk about in this group any way."

"A little bit," said Lois.

"What makes you anxious?" asked Jackie.

"Alice in Wonderland," said Kevin.

Everybody laughed. No one seemed to know whether Kevin really meant what he said or was simply being silly.

"How does Alice in Wonderland make you feel anxious?" asked Jackie. "I thought that story made children feel happy."

"Maybe it's when Alice meets the hookah smoking caterpillar," said Kevin seriously. "I think some 1960s group wrote a song about that story."

"It was Jefferson Airplane that wrote a song about Alice in Wonderland," said Jim. "I think it's called 'White Rabbit.'"

"That's very interesting," said Jackie succinctly. "I like music from the 1980s the most myself. Bangles, The Go-Go's, Bananarama, David Bowie."

"I'm late for a very important date," said Kevin.

"Meeting new people can make me anxious," responded Paisley. "Especially at a big party."

"I know what you mean, dude," said Kenneth. "I hate big parties. They make my anxiety level go up even if it doesn't look that way on the outside. I feel that way on the inside."

"Well, why don't we do a little role playing?" suggested Jackie. "How does that sound?"

"Okay," said Lois.

"I thought of something," said Paisley. "How about me asking Jim – no, Carlos – out? How would you like to go out on a date with me, Carlos?"

"What do you mean? I'm not that way," said Carlos angrily. "That's an insult."

"It's a sin," said Deanna.

"Yes, it is supposed to be a sin," agreed Carlos. "I don't know about homosexuals."

"The bible says it's a sin," said Deanna. "Man with man, woman with woman is a sin. There's a woman in my apartment building. She looks that way and talks that way."

"The Bible says it's an abomination, men with men," Roberta said.

"I don't know why anyone would choose to be gay," said Deanna. "It's terrible. I could never be that way."

"That's funny," joked Mary. "Because everyone here thinks you look like a dyke."

"Fuck you!" yelled Deanna.

"Please don't use words like that," said Jackie.

"Alright, I'm sorry," said Mary.

"You can all go to hell!" shouted Deanna, as she left the room. "I'll talk to you later white bitch!" she shouted pointing at Mary.

Deanna slammed the door really hard as she went out of the room.

"What was that all about?" asked Lois fearfully.

"Oh, thank God! She really left the room," said Mary. "I hate that big dyke."

"Nobody choses to be gay. Did you choose to be heterosexual?" said Paisley.

"I never thought of it that way before," said Roberta. "I love gay people. I just don't like what they do."

"I think people could be born that way," said Jackie. "But I'm not an expert on that subject."

"I really don't care about it that much anymore," said Mary. "Paisley is a perfectly nice guy."

"It doesn't matter to me if Paisley is gay or not," said Jim. "There are a lot of gay men in Buddhism. I'm perfectly comfortable with it."

"Thank you for saying that," said Paisley.

"People are afraid if you're different," said Tracy, a twenty-year-old black girl. "Either someone is gay or not isn't important to me. My favorite Uncle Ted is gay."

"It doesn't bother me either," said Lois. "I like Paisley no matter what he is."

"Thank you, Lois," said Paisley. "That means a lot to me."

"I love you Paisley," said Roberta. "I pray that you will change. I think if someone prays really hard that they can change."

"I love you too Roberta," said Paisley. "But I really don't want to change Roberta. I'm all right just as I am. Just pray that I stay healthy the way I already am."

"Okay Paisley," said Roberta. "But still feel funny about it."

Roberta was a pleasant 40-year-old lady with a light complexion. She once told everyone that her mother was white, and her father was black. She said her husband did not really care about that. He thought that she was beautiful inside.

"In my country people like Paisley are sometimes put into jail," said Mark, a brown eyed man in his thirties. "I don't know if there are any gay men in Turkey."

"Well, this isn't Turkey, Mark," explained Jackie. "This is the United States of America and homosexuality isn't illegal here."

"In some countries in Europe," added Paisley, "gay people can actually get married."

"Why would a man want to marry another man?" asked Roberta. "Marriage is supposed to be between a man and a woman."

"That sounds like what Arnold Schwarzenegger said in California," said Paisley. "Two gay people want to get marred for the same reason as two heterosexual people, because they are in love."

"I don't understand that," said Roberta. "It is so weird, women having sex with other women."

"What about Christine Jorgensen?" said Lois.

"That person is not the same thing as homosexuals," said Jackie. "Most gays are happy as they already are I think."

Paisley was just about to say the same thing, and then Jackie said it instead of him. Paisley realized that he had opened the proverbial can of worms with the subject of homosexuality. He wasn't really surprised by anything anyone had said, because he had heard similar statements from different people during the forty-five years of his life. Jim and the counselor Jackie's being supportive of him made this program seem much more tolerable to Paisley.

There were several issues that he normally avoided. One was abortion even though some people were in favor of a woman's right to choose. Gay marriage was another issue he knew that religious people at Campbell Care would get upset about. He avoided discussing rape and incest because some women and one man admitted to having experienced it. They probably suffered from post-traumatic stress disorder. He did not touch some people there, because they may have been abused. He only touched those who touched him. These were topics to be left alone.

The only people who touched Paisley were Mary, Tim, and Jim. Mary and Tim would often say "I love you" as they hugged him.

Sometimes they would even kiss him on the cheek. But what he really liked was to be touched by Jim. A jolt of electricity would pass though Paisley's body even if Jim just brushed past him accidentally in the hallway. Once in a while, Jim would embrace him, if he said he was feeling unloved. This was wonderful. Although Jim's full brown lips looked so appealing, Paisley knew that just one kiss could completely destroy his friendship with Jim.

One moment of pleasure Paisley could get from kissing Jim and saying "I love you" was not worth losing Jim's friendship. Jim was not the first heterosexual man with whom Paisley had been in love. He had a crush on his science teacher in seventh grade and knew somehow not to tell anyone.

While Paisley was daydreaming, he ignored what everyone was saying. He remembered where he really was when Jackie spoke again.

"I think we have discussed this subject enough," said Jackie. "Is there anything else anyone would like to talk about before this group is over?"

"I should never call Paisley a fairy, a fruit, a homo, or a faggot," said Lois.

"Lois, we tell you at Campbell Care not to use ugly words like that," said Jackie. "Keep it PG rated here."

"Yes, I remember gardenias and lilac," said Lois. "And also rhododendrons. Do you like rhododendrons Jackie?"

"I'm really not sure what they look like, Lois."

"They're big purple flowers with succulent tropical kind of leaves," explained Paisley. "My mother used to have a rhododendron bush back in Connecticut, when Alan worked for us."

"Okay I see," answered Jackie. "Have a good day everyone."

The buzzer, which sounded like an alarm clock, went off.

"You too," said Mary. "I'm sorry I got her mad."

"Please don't do that ever again, Mary," said Jackie. "She is really sensitive about her appearance."

"Who is Alan?" asked Jim. "You've never mentioned him before."

"He was my mother's gardener," said Paisley. "I can explain that another time."

"Oh my god," said Jim. "You're blushing."

Paisley touched his own face.

"You're right, Jim. My face feels very warm."

Chapter 6

Every holiday someone at Campbell Care liked to decorate the APR. They would do so with hearts on Valentine's Day, bunnies for Easter, Halloween pumpkins, and Thanksgiving pilgrims. Of course, at Christmas they usually set up a tree. It was always an artificial one. A real one would probably have been too expensive. One of the people who often organized the cheerful holiday decorating was Paisley's counselor, Eddy Aiken.

Eddy Aiken was a very handsome, and very exotic looking man. He was also the only openly gay counselor at Campbell Care. This made him and Paisley bond with each other more strongly than Paisley ever did with his former counselors. If Mr. Aiken were not Paisley's counselor, he would have asked him out on a date months before. However, it was strictly prohibited by Campbell Care to socialize with any counselor outside of program. It was considered almost as unethical as a high school teacher dating one of his or her pupils.

This time the holiday was Christmas. In home group, the first group period after morning announcements, everybody at Campbell Care gathered in their assigned rooms with their assigned counselors. Mr. Aiken's group was in room eleven. Room 11 was a large L-shaped room. There were chairs lining three walls and there were two separate doorways. There was also a gray file cabinet and a white bookcase near one of the doors. The chairs were all different looking and mismatched colors as well.

"Some of the groups are going to do something to decorate Campbell Care for Christmas," said Eddy. "I'm going to have us do the doors in here and in the APR."

"What are we going to do to the door?" asked Kenneth, who was Paisley's best friend except for Jim.

"I got some wrapping paper and bows to put on the doors."

Paisley and other people in Mr. Aiken's group covered the two doors in room 11 with Christmas wrapping paper. Then they taped a red bow onto each door, making them look like large presents. It was very festive and attractive.

"Now that we've done these doors it's time to go to the APR and decorate those doors too," said Eddy.

Mr. Aiken went into the APR with Kenneth, Paisley, Violet, Tyrone, and Karen. Paisley did not care that he was the only white person in Mr. Aiken's home group. Most of the patients at Campbell Care were African American. They were several Spanish patients, one Turkish man, and only two Asian patients. Annie and Lois were the only Jewish patients, although the owners of Campbell Care were a married Jewish couple. Just about every kind of person was represented by the staff and patients at Campbell Care. It matched the diverse community of Orange, New Jersey where Campbell Care itself was located.

There were seven doors in the APR to be decorated. Two went to the chart room where the notebooks containing the psychiatric charts of all the patients at Campbell Care were kept. Only the staff had access to these locked doors. Four doors were for four of the twelve counselors who worked at Campbell Care. One door was for the office of the assistant director of Campbell Care, a pleasant forty-five-year-old white lady named Cynthia. She was a tall thin woman with long brown hair. A set of double doors that had little windows led into Room One, right next to the Cynthia's office. They were the only doors left undecorated, because nobody was allowed to conceal the windows under wrapping paper.

There was a fake Christmas tree with blue and white lights between Room One and the wide ramp way leading to the kitchen window. This window had a counter which was where people went to get lunch and breakfast. Across from the gray kitchen door was the gray door to room 1A. Next to that was the door to the art therapist, Lisa's office. Another plain gray door next to Lisa's office led to the staff bathroom. Unlike the other bathrooms for the patients, it had a bathtub and shower in it.

Paisley and Karen decorated the first door of the chart room with red Christmas paper that had green hollies printed on it.

"We better put more tape along the bottom of the door," said Paisley.

"Okay," said Karen.

She was a nice forty-year-old black woman with hair pulled back into a small ponytail.

"I'll put more tape there," she said, kneeling in front of the door.

"What are you planning to do for Christmas?" asked Paisley, because Christmas was just six days away.

"Oh, nothing much," replied Karen sadly. "I'm just going to hang around the boarding home. What are you doing?"

"I'm going to visit my brother and sister-in-law Argyle and Candace Jubilee, and my nephew and niece."

"You're lucky you have somewhere to go."

"Yeah, I know."

"My parents are both dead and my sister Angela died from an overdose of heroin."

"That's terrible. I'm sorry."

"Shit happens. I told her to say away from that junk. She did not listen to me."

He thought he saw tears fall down Karen's face. She turned away and wiped her eyes on the sleeve of her red blouse.

Paisley realized that many mentally ill people were estranged from their families. A lot of mentally ill people were rejected by their families who did not understand or tolerate their illness. For example, Jim's own children never visited him when he was an inpatient at Greystone. Even now they only contacted him on his birthday or other holidays. This kind of estrangement from their relatives caused many patients at Campbell Care to be depressed about the holidays. They could turn to each other for solace when family fell short of caring enough.

Everyone talked about the bittersweet memories of holidays past. They recalled the gentle days when they still believed in Santa Claus, surrounded by families festooned with kind words and glittering presents. They had a real pine tree with a string of lights and pretty ornaments. Mental illness had not entered their childhood yet like a crystal prism that distorts feelings instead of beams of light.

This present holiday would be difficult for patients who were M.I.C.A., which meant "mentally ill chemical abusers." They might remember how holidays are laced with alcoholic drinks like Christmas eggnog with rum, or champagne on New Year's Eve. This might trigger them to imbibe liquor themselves or use recreational drugs to enhance their enjoyment of Christmas or New Year's Eve.

Paisley was glad that he himself had no issues with alcoholism like his father. His mother's brother had also been an alcoholic. His mother had told him how his drunken behavior had often blighted family holidays.

"Yo, Paisley," said Kenneth. "Your ride is here."

"Eddy I have to leave now, because I have my individual therapy session."

"Okay Paisley," said Eddy. "Thanks for your help."

"See you later, man."

"Okay Kenneth."

Every Wednesday, Paisley had an appointment with a psychotherapist for individual therapy. He was taken there by Reliable Van. This was the same company that took him to and from his apartment for the three days a week that he attended his program. However, he did not have Gabby as his driver, but a younger African American man named Victor. He dropped Paisley off at 10 am. for his 10:30 am. appointment at a nondescript four story office building in Livingston, New Jersey.

Paisley walked down the wide hallway to the office where his appointment was. He did some word finds to pass the time in the little lobby of New Jersey Psychiatric Group. Just before 10:30 Paisley's therapist, Allen Parker entered the room.

"Hello Paisley. I'll be with you in just a moment," said Mr. Parker.

About ten minutes later Mr. Parker opened a wooden door and said, "You can come in now, Paisley."

He had unlocked the doorway leading to the four therapy rooms.

Paisley went into room number one and lay down on the couch, while Mr. Parker sat in a comfortable leather chair. There was a small round table next to the chair with a white landline telephone on it.

"I thought I'd tell you about my Christmas holidays."

"Okay, Paisley, proceed."

"Well Campbell Care has a big feast on December twenty-first, with turkey, collard greens, macaroni and cheese, cranberry sauce. Sharon the cook there baked a diabetic sweet potato pie. It was delicious."

"I can imagine so. Do they call that 'soul food'?"

"Yes, that's soul food. Some of the patients at Campbell Care are from the South."

"So, they're not all from New Jersey, are they?"

"No, they're not."

"Why don't you tell me about last Christmas. Was it a typical Christmas for you?"

"Yes, it was. Anyway, on the twenty fourth I took Amtrak from Newark to Old Saybrook, Connecticut. My brother Argyle always buys my train ticket for me."

"That's very generous of him."

"I arrived there about three o'clock. My brother Argyle met me at the station."

"We went to Guildford, which is a little town in Connecticut. My brother took me to McDonald's for a lunch at the drive thru window."

"McDonald's? Isn't there anything better than that there?"

"Well, we were in a hurry. Then he parked his Toyota on the Boston Post Road, where most of the stores are located. He gave me some cash and I went shopping. I went into stores while he walked outside. I first when to Crabtree and Evelyn. Then I went to a gift store called Jolly's and I bought some more stocking suffers. I went into Bells and Bows and bought a kaleidoscope and lollipops and other things. Next, I went to Starbuck's and I got two more stocking stuffers. By that time, I had enough stuff. I walked back to the car and Argyle drove us home."

"That's a lot of shopping."

"Yes, it was. I spent around a hundred dollars on just stocking snuffers. I'm always in charge of the stockings every Christmas."

"Does that bother you?"

"Not really. I actually do buy a few things with my own money weeks before."

"Is there anything in this therapy that bothers you?" asked Mr. Parker solemnly holding his hands together as if in prayer.

"No, no, to both questions no. I remember how my mother used to take care of the stockings years ago. I went shopping with her a few times. That's how she showed me what kind of things make good stocking stuffers. Now that she's dead, I've taken over that duty."

"What did she die from?"

"A heart attack. She was a heavy smoker and diabetic like me. But she took insulin. I take pills. She had three of her toes amputated months before she died."

"Her equilibrium was probably affected by that. Do you miss her?"

"Less and less as the years go by. Now when I do the stocking shopping, I think of her and what she would have bought. That inspires my holiday spirit I guess."

"So, you are taking her passing in stride."

"Yes. We went to my brother and sister in law's house in Guilford. It's a big old house that they bought after my sister-in-law Candace's Aunt Betty died. It has six bedrooms, a library, a kitchen, a pantry, a sunroom and three bathrooms. The original part of house was built in the late 1700s."

Paisley was surprised by two things about Mr. Parker. First of all, it was his pen having the name of his family's funeral home on it. Second was the fact that Mr. Parker remembered what Paisley said even though he never took notes. Paisley had been seeing Mr. Parker for three years and was amazed that he never forgot anything really important. He was not only endowed with handsome Irish looks but also an amazing mind.

"Christmas Eve we had chicken and mash potatoes made fresh by Candace. That night I stuffed the stockings. My father's grandmother knitted mine and my brother's. My mother's sister, my Aunt Audrey knitted the ones for my niece and nephew."

"You have nice relatives."

"I got a DVD and $400 for Christmas. Christmas dinner was roast beef, sweet potatoes, mashed cauliflower, salad and rolls. It was delicious. My sister-in-law is an excellent cook and an excellent reporter. I think of her as the first lady of journalism. She works at a newspaper in Manhattan."

"How are your niece and nephew doing?"

"My niece Rebecca is at Harvard and my nephew Thomas is at New York University, studying music. He plays the piano and the guitar. He played some Christmas music on their piano while I was there. My father, brother and nephew all played piano."

"How was your holiday in general?"

"It was fine. Thank you for asking."

Mr. Parker looked at his gold watch on his left wrist.

"I'm afraid our time is up for today."

"Okay, Mr. Parker. I'll see you next Wednesday."

Paisley rose from the couch and left the office. He went down the hallway. He waited in front of the building where there was a covered doorway. Because the driver from Reliable Van was late, he took him directly home instead of going back to Campbell Care. After he got home, Paisley lay down on his twin bed and took a long nap. He was luckier than he usually thought he was.

All he really wanted was to find somebody to love. He remembered a quote from his Latin class in high school: "Amor vincit omnia." In other words, "Love conquers all."

Chapter 7

Often Paisley found going to a mental health program like Campbell Care could be as challenging as going to a job. Other times it felt as if he were going to school, that each group was a class and that the counselors were teachers. However, unlike school, there was never any homework. Just as he felt like taking a day off the weekends would come and rescue him.

Once a month, Paisley would go to Kenneth's house with his roommate Jeffrey. It was decided to do so during the first weekend after getting his disability check on the third of the month. He had asked Jim if he wanted to join them. Jim however preferred just to go to New York City with Paisley to see a movie every few weeks because he did not like board games.

Paisley and Jeffrey always went on Sundays to Kenneth's house, because Kenneth would visit his sister in Irvington, New Jersey on Saturdays. When they did go to Kenneth's place, they would often be driven there in an Easter Seals van by a middle-aged lady from Bermuda named Dorie. Every Monday, Wednesday, Thursday, and Sunday Dorie worked as a house coordinator at the apartment where Paisley and Jeffrey lived. She was there on mornings only on Sunday. Every other day she worked from 4 pm to 8 pm.

In his Prado Museum tote bag Paisley had placed the Scrabble, and the Yahtzee games. Yahtzee was supposed to be to dice what poker was to cards. Paisley had been playing Yahtzee since he was about seven years old. It had been an entertaining way for him to improve his math skills, because it involved addition in every single turn that he had.

"Okay, I'm ready to go," said Paisley to Dorie at noon on a Sunday morning.

Dorie, Jeffrey, and Paisley walked down the two flights of wooden stairs past the apartment on the first floor. They exited the building down the stoop to the short driveway. The tenants on the first floor were not mental health consumers in Easter Seals housing. They were regular people from the Dominican Republic.

"Could you get the garage door please, Jeffrey?" asked Dorie.

"Okay."

They got into the pigeon gray van and drove to Kenneth's house in Belleville, New Jersey, off of Belleville Avenue. It took about fifteen minutes to get there going along a two-lane road that wound its way through Branch Brook Park. During the spring, Branch Brook Park was full of cherry trees, whose ethereal blossoms were many different shades of pink.

"Have a good time, guys," said Dorie, as Jeffrey and Paisley got out of the van.

"See you tomorrow," said Paisley.

Jeffrey and Paisley walked down the little sidewalk outside of Kenneth's house. Paisley ascended the two steps up to the front door and pressed the white button of the doorbell. Moments later the wooden front door opened, and Kenneth appeared.

"Yo dudes, come in. Did Dorie drive you here?"

"Yes, she did," responded Paisley as he entered the carpeted living room.

Jeffrey closed the front door. He and Paisley went through the living room and into the dining room. They sat in two wooden chairs. Paisley removed the Yahtzee box and placed it on the blue tiled table. He put the tote bag with the Scrabble game in it onto a small wooden table in the dining room. This table was below the flight of stairs which led to the second floor of Kenneth's house.

On the second floor were three bedrooms and a full bathroom. The house had a huge kitchen off of the dining room. Another flight of stairs led down to the finished basement. There was an open space with an exercise bicycle and a half bathroom. In the far corner there were a washer and dryer, saving the residents from having to go to a laundromat.

Paisley took the top off of the cardboard box, which contained the Yahtzee game and placed it on the left side of the table. He removed the Yahtzee pad. He ripped off three individual score sheets for each of them. Kenneth removed the blue plastic Yahtzee cup and placed five red dice into it.

"We each need to pick one dice," said Paisley as he handed Kenneth and Jeffrey their own score sheets.

"Therefore, we can see who goes first," said Jeffrey.

Jeffrey picked a one, Kenneth picked a four and Paisley picked a six.

"So first goes Jeffrey. Then Kenneth. Then last but not least me."

Paisley removed three pens from the Yahtzee box. They each usually kept their own score. Paisley was very familiar with the rules of Yahtzee. He had frequently played it with his two older brothers. They had spent many hours playing board games during their summer vacations at their great grandmother's house in a small resort town called Guildford, Connecticut.

Kenneth did his three rolls of the dice and got a small straight.

"Do you want me to order the pizza now?" asked Kenneth.

"Yes, please do," said Paisley. "I didn't have any breakfast yet to save room for our pizza."

Kenneth went upstairs to his bedroom for about ten minutes to order two pepperoni pizzas and two two-liter bottles of diet soda. He always did this when they had a game day together.

"Let me see what I need," said Paisley.

He rolled three fives. Two more rolls and he had five fives. Five of a kind was called a 'Yahtzee.'

"What luck!" exclaimed Jeffrey. "I have a feeling you're going to win this one."

"I ordered our usual," said Kenneth descending the staircase, "They said about 30 minutes."

Kenneth sat down. He wore his favorite black shirt.

"What happened at program on Friday?" asked Kenneth.

He rolled his turns. He ended up with four fours and a two.

"That's four of a kind."

"Where should I begin?" said Paisley. "We got paid at noon, so that people will stay at least through the morning. My check was for $1.80."

"That's why I don't work in the workshop," said Jeffrey as he rolled the dice. "It's a real waste of time."

"They pay peanuts," said Kenneth "But it keeps some of the patients from being impatient."

"Yes, it keeps them also from being in patients at the hospital too," quipped Paisley.

"Most patients have everything else except for patience with the staff," added Kenneth.

All three of them laughed happily.

"I missed three days of work," added Paisley. "That's why I got so little money. Jim did the flours without me then."

"I had 'life skills,'" said Jeffrey. "Which we discussed dealing with a friend who betrays us. Then I had 'poetry therapy' with Holly and we talked about a couple of poems that she printed off of the Internet. Then we talked about what a home is."

"What a home is? What do you mean?"

"Is home just a place like a house or is it a state of mind?"

"I don't know. I think it's a little of both. A house is just a building, like this place I'm living in with Project Live, man."

They kept playing while talking.

"But it's the feeling of comfort and serenity that makes a house into a home," Paisley.

"Is that how you feel at Easter Seals?" asked Kenneth.

"Full house," said Jeffrey. "Two twos and three ones."

"Yes, that's how I feel about Easter Seals. First, I lived in West Orange. Then in North Newark with Jeffrey," replied Paisley. "Jeffrey is a great roommate. He doesn't even snore."

The doorbell rang. Kenneth answered the door. He got the two pizzas and Jeffrey grabbed the two-liter bottles of diet coke. Kenneth placed the pizza on the side table. Jeffrey put one of the two soda bottles onto the table.

He put the second bottle into one of the shiny white refrigerators in the kitchen. He brought 3 glasses and three plates for everyone from one of the kitchen cupboards. They got their pizza slices and soda then resumed the Yahtzee game.

"Whose turn is it?" asked Kenneth.

"Yours."

Kenneth shook the blue cup and rolled five sixes in all.

"Yahtzee! I got this one, dudes!"

"What do you mean?" said Jeffrey. "Paisley got a Yahtzee too."

"Okay, so how do you know he doesn't snore?"

"His bedroom is right next to mine. I once woke up to get a drink of water and I stood next to Jeffrey's door. I couldn't hear a peep."

"I didn't know that until you said it now," said Jeffrey with surprise.

"Yes, and thank God we don't share a bedroom, like I did in the boarding home."

"Oh shit! I hated those stupid boarding homes," agreed Jeffrey. "I got assaulted by someone at the last one where I lived."

"I'll take this," said Paisley. "Three threes is just what I needed. Now I think I'll get my bonus."

Whenever a player got 63 or more points on the top section of the score sheet, he or she would then be entitled to 35 extra points. That number of points could mean that someone could win that game. Players played six complete games. The winner was determined by adding up the entire score of all six games in that tournament.

"How the hell did you get assaulted?" asked Kenneth.

"There was this really weird guy I shared a room with. His name was Tom Jones."

"Oh no!" said Paisley. "You mean that guy from partial hospital at East Orange General Hospital?"

"Yes, I certainly do. He's the light skinned black guy that everyone said looked Hispanic."

While Jeffrey told his story, they continued playing their game.

"He once asked me out on a date."

"What! Who asked you out on a date?" said Kenneth.

"I didn't know he was like that," said Jeffrey. "Any way he and me had an argument about some money he owed me. And then out of nowhere, he punched me in the face."

Because it was warm in Kenneth's house, Paisley sipped some soda from his glass. He knew that Tom Jones was strange, but he never thought he could be violent.

"This pizza is delicious as always," said Paisley, as he put down a small straight for 30 points.

A small straight was four numbers in cardinal order like one, two, three, and four. It could also be two, three, four, and five, or three, four, five, and six on the dice.

"I'm sorry," said Paisley. "Tom Jones and you have a big fight?"

"Yes, and he hit me right on my nose. When I touched my face, there was blood coming out of my nose. Tom ran out of the room and out to the street. I told Mrs. Hemingway about it."

"Did you call the police?" asked Kenneth.

"Mrs. Hemingway, she's the lady that runs that boarding home. She calls the police and I gave them a statement."

Kenneth rolled the dice three times, as each player did during one of his turns. He ended up with two twos, a three, a five and a six. To get three of a kind he would have needed three similar dice. If he only put down two twos, instead of waiting for three of them, he would be short one two to get the needed three for ensuring the 35-point bonus.

"Damn it! This is nothing," said Kenneth.

"Put zero on Yahtzee," said Paisley. "You need to get three of the upper section. Three ones, twos, threes, fours, fives, and sixes to add up to 63 points. The minimum to get your bonus."

"That's what I'd do," said Jeffrey.

"I don't need your advice dudes," sneered Kenneth.

"Well then fuck you," said Paisley jokingly and very low.

"Listen if anyone's going to do the fucking it's me, man," said Kenneth. "I'm the top of the heap."

"What do you mean by that?" asked Jeffrey. "I thought you were celibate."

"Alright, I'll put zero on Yahtzee," said Kenneth.

They all three laughed.

"I'm getting another slice of pizza," said Paisley.

"Could you get me another one too?" asked Kenneth.

"Why don't I get another one for all of us," added Paisley. "You lazy bum."

Paisley brought one of the boxes of pizza to the table. Both Jeffrey and Kenneth helped themselves to a slice each. Paisley put one on his own plate. It was a plain white plate, which was part of the dishware that Project Live provided for its tenants.

"Yeah so, what happened to Tom Jones?" asked Kenneth.

"I think they moved him to another boarding home after that."

"That's the least they could do," said Paisley. "You're such a nice guy Jeffrey. You deserve better treatment than that. Some of those boarding homes are real hell holes."

"I know what you mean," agreed Kenneth. "That's why I am glad to be in this house owned by Project Live."

"I had to share a room with two other guys at my boarding home. It was almost like being back in a dorm room at college," said Paisley. "Now at Easter Seals I have my own bedroom."

"Where did you go to college?" asked Jeffrey. "Was it in Connecticut?"

"No, it was in New York State. The State University of New York at Albany. Because my father lived in that state, I got a reduced tuition."

"I just rolled four sixes and a five," said Jeffrey. "That's 29 points for four of kind. Isn't that right?"

"That's the best four of kind you can get," said Paisley. "The only thing better than that is five sixes, which is also

50 points for a Yahtzee. Two Yahtzees and you get an extra 100 points."

"I know that," said Kenneth "Is that some kind of message here? I get Yahtzees but Mr. College Grad gets squat."

"College is knowledge. Yahtzee is all about luck," said Paisley sarcastically. "It's not the same thing. I could buy you some books to read like the ones that college students read."

"Whatever. Are we all through?" asked Kenneth.

"Yes, we are. Now add up your total and we'll see who won."

"Jeffrey got one hundred twenty-three points. I got one hundred twenty-four points and you won with one hundred eighty-five points."

"Do you want to play another game of Yahtzee?" asked Paisley.

"I need to take a smoke break man," said Kenneth.

He got up and went to the living room. He sat down on the moss green sofa and opened a pack of cigarettes. He took a small crystal blue lighter and lit the cigarette. Paisley opened one of the windows next to the table where they had been playing Yahtzee for ventilation. Both he and Jeffrey disliked cigarette or marijuana smoke.

"You have all the time in world," said Paisley.

He poured another glassful of diet coke for himself and Jeffrey. He waited a few seconds for the bubbles to fizzle out before he took his first sip.

"If we were playing strip poker, you'd be nude by now," said Kenneth. "A nude dude. That's cool."

"What? You want me to take it off or something?"

"It's getting hot in here so take off all your clothes," sang Kenneth.

"You have a dirty mind Kenneth," said Paisley. "I want a divorce!"

"Oh yeah I remember that song," said Jeffrey. "Who sang that any way?"

"Captain and Tennille," joked Paisley. "The Village People."

"What! That song came out way after the 1970s," said Jeffrey. "You must be kidding."

"Oh, who cares," said Paisley. "I'll look that up on the internet at the Newark Public Library next time I go there."

"I didn't know that you could go online at the Public Library," said Jeffrey. "Is it free?"

"Yes, Jeffrey. You bring a photo id like your driver's license with your current address on it. They hand to you a free library card that's good for one year. The computers are on the third floor."

Paisley finished his third slice of pizza. There was one slice left. Kenneth split it in two and gave one half to Jeffrey.

They put the five red dice back into the blue plastic cup. Kenneth picked a six, Jeffrey picked a one, and Paisley picked a five. That meant that Kenneth went first, Paisley went second, and Jeffrey went last.

"Do you still have a crush on Jim?" asked Kenneth.

"You mean Jim Everett?" asked Jeffrey. "Full house."

"Yes him," said Paisley. "Yes, I still do. He said that he might move back down to South Carolina someday to be with his mother. He said that one of his brothers and sister live down south, so he would see all of them more often. I think I may ask him to move down with him."

"Are you crazy?" said Kenneth. "You'd leave all your friends up here behind and leave Campbell Care too?"

"Yes, I would, if Jim would let me."

"Do you love him that much?"

"Yes, I do. I think he is a wonderful person. He is intelligent, handsome kind to me, easy to work with when we do the flours together. The only thing I don't like about him is that he sometimes smokes."

Paisley took his turn. He rolled a small straight and wrote down the score.

"I think you're going to win this one," said Kenneth.

"I didn't know that Jim was gay," said Jeffrey.

"I thought he was straight," said Kenneth as he sipped his soda.

"He is straight, but I still love him anyway."

"You're crazy," said Kenneth. "You're gonna move with a straight man. What kind of relationship will that be?"

"So, it will be a platonic one," said Paisley. "That's fine with me."

"What does platonic mean?" asked Jeffrey as he took his turn.

"It means no sexual contact," said Paisley "We'd be celibate."

"Oh, I see now," said Jeffrey. "Two fours and three ones. That's a full house, right?"

"At the age I am at now, which is forty—."

"You don't look that old," commented Kenneth.

"He and I were both born in 1965," said Jeffrey. "My birthday is March 19 and Paisley's is September 19. I am exactly six months older than him."

"Thank you. Any way after all that I've been through and with the diseases now, I don't care much about sex anymore. So, a platonic relationship doesn't bother me. In a way, it's easier because I don't have to be performing."

"If Jim dropped his pants, I bet you'd do him," said Kenneth. "Admit it, man."

"Well, I guess so. Who knows? Maybe he will realize some day that he has latent homosexual tendencies?"

"You guess so."

"It's been so long since I last had sex that I'm not sure I know what to do anymore."

They all laughed.

"I don't think that I care about sex anymore either," said Jeffrey. "Sex is overrated any way. It's all over the TV. Love is more important."

"I'd like to take a smoke break before we continue anything else, man."

"Okay," said Paisley.

Paisley stretched his legs and went into the kitchen to get more diet coke. Jeffrey stayed in the dining room while Kenneth smoked a Marlboro cigarette in the living room.

"Do you always smoke the same brand of cigarettes?" asked Paisley "My mother always insisted on smoking only Parliament cigarettes."

"Yeah, I try to smoke only one brand," answered Kenneth. "But I can't always afford Marlboros. Sometimes I smoke el cheapo cigarettes like Waves."

"Do you want to play Yahtzee again or Scrabble?" asked Paisley.

"Yahtzee," said Jeffrey.

"We can play Scrabble later."

They played six games of Yahtzee altogether, making it a complete tournament. After they added up their total scores, Jeffrey won. Then they played a game of Scrabble which Kenneth won easily because he got the letters with the most point values like the Q and the Z. After that Kenneth called them a cab and Jeffrey and Paisley went home, talking about their pleasant Sunday.

Chapter 8

Paisley Jubilee had always had very mixed feelings about his father, partly because of his giving him an unusual name like Paisley. When he was young, he used to be teased a lot about his peculiar name. Paisley had often thought of getting his name legally changed as did his equally oddly named brothers Argyle and Plaid. Nevertheless, as they got older, they realized that having an unusual name made it easier for people to remember them.

One cause of Paisley's ambivalent feelings about his father was his alcoholism Mr. Derek Jubilee sometimes became angry and violent whenever he was intoxicated. He never took out his anger on his children. He would argue with Paisley's mother Camille instead. One time Paisley had observed an argument when his father struck his mother a couple of times. Paisley always remembered this incident, which happened before his parents' divorce. All his father ever said about it was "I'm sorry who had to see that." Paisley had never fully forgiven his father for harming his weaker mother, even after his parents finally passed away. He sometimes had nightmares about domestic violence. He feared that a male lover might snap on him some day, and so avoided alcoholic gay men.

When he had worked at a legal newspaper, Paisley had assisted a closeted female reporter in writing about the particular legal problems of gay men and lesbians. Reporting domestic violence to homophobic police officers could be complicated if the assailant was a homosexual lover.

After his parents' divorce was final, his father began dating other women besides his mother. Mr. Jubilee moved to Manhattan when Paisley was 10. Paisley remained alone with his mother in Connecticut until he was 14. When he was 11 years old, Paisley's brother Plaid went off to college and Argyle went to an exclusive boarding school paid for by an inheritance from one of his mother's maiden aunts. After his occasional visits with his father, his mother would ask him questions about his father's current girlfriend. One incident was somewhat funny.

"What was his girlfriend's name?" asked Camille, Paisley's mother.

"Bunny. Or maybe she was a bunny. I don't know."

"You mean he's now dating a Playboy bunny?"

"I guess so. What is that?"

"A Playboy bunny is a waitress at the Playboy clubs for men. Like the Playboy magazine."

"Oh yeah, now I get it, Mother."

"Your father always had an eye for the ladies, Paisley. But when his hands followed his roving eyes I asked for a divorce."

Paisley had trouble right after the divorce understanding how his father could have ever stopped loving his mother. Paisley loved both his parents and never could completely comprehend fully how they stopped loving each other. It hurt him to see the clear evidence of the end of his parents' tumultuous relationship. All of Paisley's friends would later on agree that his father was not a very good role model.

The situation was changed one night in a very dramatic way in May 1980. Paisley was still living with his mother then in a house deep in the woods of Guildford, Connecticut. His brother Argyle was visiting for a few days. This was four years after his parents' divorce.

His father came to visit. He got into a big fight with Paisley's mother. His brother Argyle and he drove away without any of Paisley's clothes. After spending the night at a friend of Argyle, Paisley's father drove Paisley to Manhattan. That was when Derek Jubilee decided that Paisley was going to live with him until Paisley went to college himself.

His father eventually settled into a monogamous relationship with a woman named Erica when Paisley moved to Manhattan in 1980. His father had tired of the previous short-term relationships with other, younger women. Many of them simply wanted him to get them a job on the television news program for which he worked during most of his career.

Erica never asked Paisley about his mother or Derek's previous relationships. Paisley was glad about that. Nevertheless, Paisley's mother Camille did ask him personal questions about his father's newest relationship. His father never asked Paisley if his mother was dating anyone.

Another thing that had irked Paisley was his father's insistence that he go to a psychiatrist when he was 15 and first began living with his father. He made Paisley go to a

Freudian children's doctor for ten grueling sessions before he was willing to end the treatment. Later on, when he was 21 Paisley was more willing to accept the idea of seeing a psychiatrist at his father's expense. Paisley felt better about himself, even though he was still not being prescribed any medications yet.

"Did I tell you that I have gone to other therapists and a psychiatrist before," Paisley asked his current psychotherapist Mr. Parker.

"No, I don't think we've ever discussed that," replied Mr. Parker adjusting his tie.

Mr. Parker always dressed very nattily during his therapy sessions with Paisley. It was as if he were working in a corporate office setting.

"Yes, I did see someone before. The first time was when I was a teenager. Then I went to one when I was 21. When I saw another one at 25 years old, he was willing to let me pay him on a sliding scale like you. At that time, I was working so my father wouldn't pay any more for my treatment. I was finally independent. I only got a $40 check on my birthday from him. And a $500 check for Christmas. He rarely gave me anything else, although I knew he could afford it."

"You sound a little upset about that."

"I was. I was always surrounded by money and my mother Camille had rich selfish friends. But I don't remember her telling me that they ever helped her out. Except that when she moved into an apartment in downtown Guilford. Her best friend's cousin owned the house it was in and charged her a very low rent."

"Well often having rich friends doesn't necessarily mean that will enrich your own life," said Mr. Parker knowingly. "Maybe your mother was too embarrassed to ask her friends for any money."

"My mother was raised by her wealthy grandparents. She probably knew nothing about food stamps or anything like that."

"I suppose so."

"And my father never really adjusted to the fact that one of his three children was a homosexual."

"You mean your older brothers are heterosexual? That is not unusual."

"I never felt very close to my father. He was never very affectionate toward any of his children. Even before I came out to him, he never showed any affection toward me. It wasn't until I was in my thirties that he would even hug me, and it was always very hesitantly."

"A lot of men have trouble showing affection, particularly toward other men," suggested Mr. Parker.

"I guess that it's homophobia."

"Paisley, I guess your father was from the old school."

"And I remember another problem with my father Derek Jubilee. When he was involved with his girlfriend Barbara, whom he got involved with after dumping Erica, he went to her son's high school graduation from an exclusive boarding school. My father did not attend my high school graduation from Thomas Academy. My mother, my father's brother, and my brother Argyle did attend though."

"I don't blame you for feeling bad about that."

Mr. Parker took a drink from a water bottle on the desk next to his chair. He never drank soda.

"And when I got accepted to Boston University, I couldn't get financial aid. They said that my father made too much money."

"It was an embarrassment of riches literally."

"But when I asked him to pay for my tuition, he refused to at first. But my mother pushed him to pay it. He let me down on many occasions."

"He does not seem like a candidate for father of the year."

"No, definitely not," said Paisley bitterly as he sipped some soda from a can of diet coke. "He probably should never have had children at all."

"I don't know about that. That's perhaps being a little too harsh."

"Well, maybe so. He did pay for my trips to London and Paris in 1992 and 1993. He was working in London for NBC news from 1992–1995. I went to visit him for two Christmases. But he told me after my lover Boris had bought planes tickets to Paris that he was not letting Boris come after all. Boris was very hurt about that."

"Your father probably couldn't handle seeing you with your lover. It would have been definite confirmation of your sexual orientation."

"I guess you are right. It was proof positive of my homosexuality. I don't think he was ever really comfortable with it. He never talked to me about sexuality of any kind, whether it was homosexuality, heterosexuality, or bisexuality. I just know that he had a subscription to Playboy magazines because I found them in his den once. I rarely saw him and my mother hug or kiss or anything while I was growing up."

"He wasn't a very good role model, as your friends said."

"No, he wasn't, and that's not all. His will got changed. He first wrote a will in 1990. In that will he left $45,000 to Argyle, Plaid, and me each. Then I got a copy from my wicked stepmother of my father's second will. She had changed his will to leave everything to my stepmother, the greedy bitch."

"I can understand why you have such mixed feeling about your father. You think that he betrayed you in many ways. He divorced your mother. He had trouble showing affection toward you."

"Do you see now why I feel about him the way I do?"

"Yes, I do. Maybe we can discuss next time trying to forgive your father."

Paisley took another sip from his can of diet coke.

"I'm afraid that our time is up."

Paisley removed from his tote bag the transportation form from Reliable Van Service. Mr. Parker had to sign it in order to prove to the van service that he had used their services to go to a medical appointment. People were not allowed to use the van service for personal matters, like going to a supermarket or a massage parlor.

"I'll see you next Wednesday. Think about your father outside of the box."

"Take care, Mr. Parker."

"Be well, Paisley."

Paisley and Kenneth walked down the long hallway to the elevator on the third floor. They walked through the lobby of the building. There was a dark blue sofa and two matching chairs, with a mahogany coffee table between them. They waited at the front driveway under a shady breezeway. There was a low brick wall decorated with a large flowerbox with festive orange and yellow marigolds inside of it. They sat on the section of this wall that was empty.

"How did your session go?" asked Kenneth as he lit a cigarette.

"It went okay. I talked about my father."

"Oh no, not him again. I barely knew my old man, dude."

About ten minutes later Gabby pulled up in a green unmarked Reliable Van Service van to take Kenneth and Paisley back to their respective and respectable homes. Kenneth lived in Belleville, New Jersey, while Paisley still lived in North Newark.

Chapter 9

Sexuality of any kind was something about which Paisley had never thought much until he was thirteen. He started growing pubic hair and masturbated for the first time to orgasm. His parents never discussed puberty or sexuality with Argyle, Plaid or him. He knew instinctively that it was an important subject to other people too.

Paisley's counselor Eddy ran the so-called Human Sexuality group. He was a perfect choice to run this group. Unlike other counselors who were embarrassed about discussing sexual matters, Eddy was quite open about his sexual orientation. He once told Paisley that he doesn't care who knows that I'm gay. He was not conservative in his thinking like others who think sex is only acceptable between a man and a woman and that they must be married. He was accepting of premarital sex and sex between consenting adults.

Eddy had different ways of getting his point across. Often they would discuss certain topics like AIDS, orgasms, avoiding sexually transmitted diseases. Occasionally Eddy would show videos. These videos dealt with issues like AIDS, HIV, HPV, intimacy, masturbation, and communication.

But what Paisley liked most of all was the group discussions. Then he would hear the true stories of real people's sex lives.

Paisley was the first one to enter the room as usual. He sat on one of the black plastic chairs with chrome legs next to a collapsible table with a simulated wood finish. About ten other people entered the plain white room. Like every other group room, this one had a ghostly white-faced clock on the wall.

"Mr. Paisley," said Roberta as she sat down next to him as she always did.

"Mrs. Roberta."

Eddy entered the room and sat down as the bell rang informing everyone that a new group had started. He was wearing very attractive and coordinated clothes as usual. He wore a leopard print shirt. He had around his neck a small St. Christopher's medal. He had a nice pair of black jeans and black loafers. He could probably have been a male model instead of a counselor.

"Before we start our discussion, I want to remind everybody that what is discussed in here is confidential," admonished Eddy. "What is said in here stays in here."

"What happens in Vegas stays in Vegas," said Mark, the Turkish man.

"Can you tell someone is gay just from looking at them?" asked Eddy.

"No, you can't," said Stan. "Paisley probably knows more about that than anyone here." Stan was a middle-aged white man with a gray hair, and a goatee. He had a nice baritone voice, which Paisley thought would be excellent for voice over work.

"Sometimes you can tell," said Mary. "But not always."

"Do I look gay, Mary?" asked Paisley.

"No, you don't," said Mary. "I didn't mean to be insulting."

"I'm not sure what it means to look gay," said Roberta. "Is that feminine?"

Roberta was a 40-year-old light-skinned woman with a small afro. She wore glasses but still had trouble seeing things. She often told Paisley "I love you," even though she was married for 14 years to a nice white man named Owen.

"No, the stereotype is that gay men are feminine, but they aren't," explained Eddy calmly. "It could mean a certain way you dress."

"Some ignorant people think that they can tell someone is gay from just looking at them," said Paisley. "Like lesbians are supposed to look butch with short hair, flannel shirts, and work boots."

"What does 'butch' mean?" asked Lois.

"A woman who looks masculine," said Eddy. "Like a man does."

"But dressing like that doesn't mean you're a lesbian. There are some who are called 'lipstick' lesbians."

"I've heard of them," said Mary. "Although I've never met one."

"My cousin Jessica is one," said Paisley "and she's still a bitch."

"Your cousin is gay too?" asked Mary.

"Yes, she is. My aunt has had problems dealing with her being gay."

"You still don't talk to Jessica after ten years?" asked Mary.

"We had a big fight after aunt died and she won't reconcile with me," said Paisley. "We've always had a love hate relationship."

"This may be a good time to change gears a little," said Eddy "What does it take to have a good relationship with someone?"

"Lots of sex. Chris used to do it with me every night," said Annie. "He wore me out because he was big and black."

Annie was a large white woman who was fifty years old. She dyed her hair black and always wore red lipstick. She sometimes complained that she could never find a nice Jewish man to love her.

"I haven't had sex in fifteen years," said Lois. "I don't need a man to make me happy. I don't want a boyfriend who is not Jewish anyway."

"Fifteen years! I could never go even fifteen weeks without having it," said Annie. "Sometimes they pay me ten dollars to do it, the guys in my boarding house."

"Do you use condoms every time you have sex?" asked Eddy.

"No, I don't," answered Annie. "Some guys don't like to wear them."

"You have no self-respect," said Mary. "My body is a temple. I would never let no man use me especially for only ten dollars."

"You should be more careful Annie," said Eddy. "In this day and age there are lots of diseases you could catch. Some might lead to cervical cancer."

"I never thought of that," responded Annie. "Sometimes I need money really bad and guys will pay me to do it."

"You're just being like a cheap prostitute," said Mary. "It's so pathetic."

"Ten dollars is nothing. Real prostitutes charge like $20 or more," said Mark. "I use them sometimes."

"They probably couldn't afford that much in my boarding home," said Annie.

"You shouldn't be doing this in the first place Annie," said Paisley "That's not a good relationship."

"That brings me back to the original question of what makes a good relationship," said Eddy.

"Trust," said Jim in a striped shirt. "You have to trust the other person, or you can't have anything with them. That includes friends."

Jim looked at Paisley.

"Thank you, Jim."

"If you can't trust them then they might be cheating on you," said Mary.

"You have to trust them because sometimes people lie about their HIV status," said Paisley. "They say they're HIV negative, when they're really HIV positive. Plus there are other diseases like syphilis, herpes, HPV, and gonorrhea."

"It's important to protect yourself from diseases," said Eddy. "But you shouldn't let that stop you from having a relationship with somebody."

"You also shouldn't fall in love with someone who is straight," said Paisley.

Many people laughed including Jim. Paisley was sitting next to him as he often did when they were in the same group together. It was part of his comfort zone.

"You need to have good communication between you and other people," added Jim. "That's important even if you're just friends."

"I'm glad that you mentioned that," said Eddy. "What relationships are there besides boy girl relationships or romantic relationships?"

"A mother and a child," said Annie. "A counselor and a patient like here at Campbell Care."

"Are there any restrictions on relationships?" asked Eddy.

"Yes, there are," said Paisley. "A husband shouldn't beat his wife."

"Was there domestic violence in your home?" asked Roberta.

"Yes, there was, especially when my father was drunk," said Paisley. "He was like another person when he was drunk."

"Domestic violence was in my family too," said Mary. "Both my parents were alcoholics, and they would beat us too, as kids. Me and my brother."

"No child should have to go through that," said Eddy. "Or molestation either."

"I was molested by my uncle," said Annie who started crying. "It was terrible."

Mary got up and sat next to Annie. She held her hands, and said, "Don't cry Annie."

"I can't help it."

"It's okay. It's okay," said Mary maternally.

"How old were you when this happened?" asked Eddy.

"I was seven. Seven to fourteen. I don't want to talk about it anymore it's too upsetting," said Annie. "I was brought up to be a good Jewish girl."

Everyone stopped talking for a few minutes.

"Maybe you should discuss it in women's group," suggested Eddy.

"That's a good idea," said Mary. "Discuss it tomorrow in women's group Annie."

"Okay," said Annie. "But I might cry again."

"That's alright Annie," said Eddy. "Sometimes we need to cry."

"Everyone cries at some time or another," said Jim. "Even men cry too, like when their wives decide to divorce them."

"So obviously what Annie, Mary and Paisley had gone through was not what makes a good relationship. People need to respect your boundaries and not lay their hands on you," explained Eddy. "Particularly when you're a defenseless child."

"A good relationship means having something in common with the other person," said Mary.

"It doesn't matter if you're gay, straight or bisexual, a man or a woman. The same problems come up: sex, jealousy and more. I have talked to all kinds of people, and I've decided that to be true in my forty-four years on this planet," said Paisley.

"You don't look forty-four to me Paisley," said Lois winking at him. "I still think that you are handsome."

"Well of course you'll fight over these," said Mary. "It doesn't matter what race you are either. You need the same things to have a good relationship."

"And we established that these things are trust, good communication, and having similar interests," said Eddy. "What else is there?"

"Honesty," said Lois. "No one loves a liar. I would never date a liar, criminal or a jerk."

"Very good Lois," said Eddy.

"Respect," said Jim succinctly.

Jim had always been a man of few words. Paisley realized this often, knowing him for four years. When he did speak, he always said something that you wanted to know.

"Someone who's a good listener," said Paisley. "Like Jim. He may not say much but I know that he is paying attention to what is being said around him."

Paisley wondered if Jim listened between the lines of his statements about how much he cared about him and how much he would miss him if he really moved to South Carolina. Jim had said that the boarding home where he lived was going to be sold. He would have to move, probably to his widowed mother's home in a little town in South Carolina.

"Thank you," said Jim.

"You're very welcome," said Paisley.

"If you don't respect someone, how could you have a relationship with him?" asked Roberta "It's impossible. My husband respects me."

"You have to love yourself before you can love anyone else," said Eddy. "Isn't that true?"

"Yes, it is," said Paisley. "I often wonder how much some people whom I have known loved themselves. They're the ones who were alcoholics."

"Is having sex with men for ten dollars a shot loving yourself?" asked Eddy.

"No, it isn't," agreed Annie. "I see your point now. I won't do it anymore."

"Do you really mean that?" asked Eddy.

"Yes, I do," said Annie. "I guess my childhood experience makes me have low self-esteem. I don't want to be a whore."

"That's very possible, Annie," said Eddy. "A lot of abused people feel that way. And that may be why those people you knew, Paisley, were alcoholics."

"I'll talk about it in Women's group," said Annie. "Maybe I'll feel less embarrassed then."

"Good," said Eddy. "That way you can talk about it in more detail."

"A good relationship, even if it's just friends and not at all sexual, is someone you're comfortable with," said Paisley. "Someone you can be yourself with and not have to hide your real self from."

"I see. So, in other words you can be out with him," said Eddy. "Jim you don't care that he's gay?" asked Eddy.

"No, it doesn't matter to me," said Jim. "They are some gays in Buddhism too."

"It doesn't matter to us either," said Mary. "You can choose whatever lifestyle you want. I still love you Paisley. As a friend I mean."

Mary kept on twirling a lock of her gray hair when she said that. She was nervous when anyone discussed sexual matters.

"I don't think you choose to be gay or straight," said Eddy. "But you can choose whether to come out of the closet or not. I think you could be born that way."

"I heard it might be genetic," said Paisley.

"I never thought of it that way," said Mary. "So, there might be a gay gene?"

"Yes," said Paisley. "I guess it could be in your DNA, but I'm not totally sure of that."

"That's weird. So, someone could tell from a blood test if you're gay or not?" asked Mary.

"Well, that's a good question. I really don't know if the technology is that advanced yet, or not," said Paisley. "It just makes me wonder why it matters so much to people like my father whether someone is gay or not."

"People are fascinated by things that they don't understand," said Eddy.

"Or things that they are afraid of," said Roberta. "I guess I'm afraid of lesbians because they might make a pass at me."

"That's disgusting," said Mary. "A woman wanting to love me."

"I've never known any dykes or queers," said Lois. "Are they really all in Greenwich Village?"

"Gay men are a threat to men and an insult to women," said Eddy.

"They are treated like aliens from another planet in a science fiction novel that I read," said Jim.

Jim had read a lot of science fiction books. They helped him to forget his mental illness. His favorite novel was called Dune.

"That's a very good analogy Jim," said Eddy. "You hit the nail on the head."

At that moment, the bell rang at Campbell Care signaling the end of that period.

"Maybe we could continue this discussion next week," suggested Eddy.

"This was a great group," said Paisley.

"Yes, it was," agreed Jim, as they left room 8. "I love you spiritually, Paisley."

"Thank you."

"But I have to admit that I used to feel like laughing whenever somebody said your name."

"Yeah, Paisley Jubilee is a weird name, I know. I used to be called 'P.J.' a lot too."

Chapter 10

There were many different therapy groups that Paisley had to attend as part of what was called his treatment plan. This was decided by Paisley and his counselor Eddy as the groups that would benefit him the most. Everyone at Campbell Care had been assigned a counselor and a treatment plan. It was revised every six months. Sometimes a trauma would happen that would send someone back into the hospital, however.

One of the therapy groups to which Paisley was assigned was called stress reduction and relaxation. This was the only group he had that had a rotating staff of different counselors. This group was scheduled Monday through Friday right before the second lunch period which ran from 12:30 pm to 1 pm.

Some counselors played soothing classical music or a jazz station on the radio. Some counselors would play relaxation tapes with breathing and stretching exercise narrated by a man with a melodious voice. Campbell Care had one counselor named Suzanna, a pretty Italian-American, lady who was 25 years old. She would conduct mental exercises for the fifteen or so people in the group. It usually took place in room 9.

Room 9 was similar to most of the other eleven rooms at Campbell Care. It was painted white and contained about 20 chairs of different styles because most of the chairs were donations. It had some decorations on the walls made by actual patients of Campbell Care. There were pictures drawn with crayons or painted with watercolors. None of them were good enough to be displayed in a public art gallery.

But what was more unusual about room 9 was its being in the section of the building that used to be part of a dance club. The ceiling had mirrored tiles, instead of plain white ones. If you looked up, you could see your reflection staring back at you. This was terrible on a bad hair day!

Suzanna handed out a list of stressors that she got from the Internet. Most of the counselors at Campbell Care used the internet as a source of information to use in therapy groups. The stressors were categorized as either major or minor ones. The first one said, "Your alarm clock not going off."

"Minor definitely minor," said Annie.

"That's happened to me a lot," said Dwayne.

He was a young black man who had excellent charming attributes. A framed portrait that Dwayne had drawn of Martin Luther King was on one of the blue walls of the APR, the all-purpose room. He was one of the few people there who actually possessed artistic ability.

"Your favorite sports team losing," said Suzanna.

"Minor," said Dwayne. "Except when my favorite team the Devils loses."

The Devils was a hockey team based in nearby Newark, New Jersey. Paisley often saw people dressed in black and red Devils shirts on the Newark light rail system coming home from hockey games. Some of the patients at Campbell Care were perplexed by the team's name being "The Devils."

"Major when the Mets lose," said Gino. "Then I might as well kill myself."

Gino was a white haired balding white man with a mustache. His large belly made him a reluctant choice to play Santa Claus when Campbell Care had their annual Christmas party in the APR. He was diagnosed as being bipolar.

"Please don't," said Suzanna.

"I was just kidding," said Gino.

"I hope so," said Suzanna. "Suicide really isn't a great thing to joke about. If I thought you were serious, I would have to inform somebody about it."

The room fell silent for a little while.

"A recent illness?"

"Major," said Mary, who rode on Paisley's van driven by Gabby. "I have had to deal with a recent illness. I sometimes bleed a little from my vagina. I hope I don't wake up one day hemorrhaging."

"Have you seen your gynecologist recently?" asked Suzanna. "Women your age should get seen regularly."

"I haven't seen one in years," said Annie.

"I have an appointment to see Dr. Coretta next Monday," said Mary merrily. "I know what to do since I reached the change of life."

"Very good," said Suzanna. "You haven't seen one in years, Annie? Do you still have your period?"

"No, I don't have a period anymore," said Annie. "My mother used to call it her 'monthly curse.'"

"You should talk about that in women's group," said Suzanna helpfully. "Maybe someone your age could give you good advice."

"Yes," said Lois. "I'm getting over a little cold. At my age it takes longer to recover, doesn't it, Paisley? At least it's not pneumonia or scarlet fever."

"I suppose so," replied Paisley. "Diabetics like me take longer to get well. My primary care physician says that I should check my glucose levels more whenever I'm sick."

"Having a cold can be a drag, I know," said Suzanna. "I also have allergies."

Suzanna sneezed right after she said that.

"Bless you!" said Annie.

"Oh God don't even let me get started on that subject," said Mary. "I'm allergic to penicillin."

"My mother was allergic to penicillin," said Paisley. "She also smoked like a chimney. Her favorite was Parliament cigarettes."

"I quit smoking three years ago," said Lois. "With the patch."

"Congratulations!" said Suzanna.

Everybody applauded after Lois's wonderful announcement. They were all glad too when she did not talk in her usual word salads. She had a compulsion to talk sometimes in lists that often-included inappropriate words. Only new patients at Campbell Care were still offended by her off color statements.

"I'm allergic to seafood like lobsters and shrimp," said Mary. "I'm allergic to strawberries and blueberries. I get hives all over my arms. It's terrible."

"My mother is also allergic to penicillin," said Suzanna, briskly. "Has anyone also experienced a recent illness? Okay, the next stressor is dealing with bureaucracy slash red tape. Surely all of you have dealt with this at one time or another. Getting food stamps, welfare. Is that major or minor?"

There was a short silence.

"Yes, that is a major one. I have definitely experienced that problem," explained Paisley. "It took me three years and three denials to get my disability from the Social Security Administration."

"What is the difference between disability and SSI?" asked Lois naively. "I get SSI, but I couldn't get disability."

"You have to have a work history in order to get disability," said Suzanna. "If you've never worked or only worked a little but off and on you can't get disability. You can only get SSI which is Supplemental Security Income."

"I get SSI," said Mary. "I get my check on the first day of every month. I have it direct deposited into my checking account. It's a lot safer than having your check sent to you in the mail."

"Yeah, it can be stolen that way," said Suzanna. "They don't like using the snail mail anymore. It is what it is."

"I get SSI," said Gino. "I used to work at Quik Chek in Kearny, New Jersey. But I got fired when I had a manic episode. I drove my car really fast with no shirt on and the radio blasting. The police arrested me and put me in Cedar Grove."

"I get disability, but I was denied at first," said Liza. "Those bitches downtown put me through the wringer."

Liza was a thirty-year-old white woman with really short, brown hair. She had a black barbed wire tattoo around her upper left arm. She also had a pierced tongue. Paisley found her intriguing and wondered if she was a lesbian.

"I had enough credits to get disability. You have to have enough work credits. For every year you worked you get four credits," said Paisley. "I worked as a live in babysitter for a cousin and had her take out my Social Security taxes. Before that I worked five years at a legal journal in Washington, D.C."

"Did you go to law school?" asked Liza. "My mother is a legal secretary so I know what assholes lawyers can be."

"Liza, please keep it PG rated here," said Suzanna. "Words like that are considered unacceptable here."

"Okay," said Liza. "I'm sorry I said 'assholes.' I mean that bad word."

Paisley and Liza laughed.

"I didn't know it was that complicated," said Mary. "So, you get four credits per year, and you need forty credits to get disability?"

"No, I never went to law school," answered Paisley. "I took a proof-reading test in order to get my job as an editorial assistant."

"How long did you live in Washington, D.C.?" asked Gino. "Because I've never even left New Jersey. Except to go to New York a few times."

"I lived there about 12 years," answered Paisley. "I still like New Jersey better though."

"You really like New Jersey?" asked Liza. "I always thought New York City would be a better place for gays than this one."

"Are you gay?" asked Mary. "I thought so but since you mentioned gays, I thought I'd ask any way."

"Yes, I am a lesbian," said Liza. "But please don't tell anyone. Well, you can tell K.D. Lang."

Liza started chuckling. Paisley doubted that most people in room understood her sarcasm in the way that he did.

"Well back to the stressors," said Suzanna "A divorce. Is that minor or major?"

"Major, I guess," said Annie. "I've never been married, but I think a divorce must feel really lousy. Especially if you have lived without sex, or wine coolers."

"You've never been married? I'm surprised someone like you hasn't been married at least once, twice three times a lady," said Liza sarcastically.

Paisley was beginning to like Liza. He thought it was refreshing that somebody at Campbell Care had a sense of humor at all.

"Yes, I know it is," agreed Paisley. "I got divorced after marrying a lesbian friend whom I had known for many years. I only married her because I was homeless. A bad idea."

"Wow, that's pretty bad," said Suzanna. "That's definitely a major stressor. Has anyone else gone through a divorce?"

"Yes, I have," said Liza. "My mother and my father got divorced when I was only three. I hardly knew my father at all. I agree with Paisley that it is a really bad thing to go through."

"I've never even been married," stated Suzanna. "So I've never been divorced. I hope when I do get married it will be forever."

"I hope so too," said Annie. "You are such a nice person that I think you deserve the best. Just like I do."

"Thank you, Annie," said Suzanna. "I hope when I do get married it lasts forever."

"Who'd want to marry someone like you?" sneered Mary. "You're so big."

"There's more of me to love," said Annie. "I think I have a beautiful body."

"Oh God not that again," said Mary. "I'm sorry I said anything now."

"Mary we're not supposed to insult anyone here," scolded Suzanna. "Campbell Care is supposed to be a supportive environment."

"Alright, Annie," said Mary. "I'm sorry."

"Well, the next stressor on this list is 'losing a friend's phone number.' I know that's happened to me. How about anyone else?"

"Yes," said Jessica. "It was really frustrating. But my son called soon afterwards, so I got back his number."

"Can't you store numbers on your phone?" asked Liza. "I have all my friends' numbers at my fingertips."

"I don't like cell phones," said Lois. "I can't understand how to use one."

"I had a similar situation," explained Paisley. "But it was a more up to date problem. I lost a friend's email address who lives in Russia. I had to call his parents in

Michigan to get back his email address. My roommate Jeffrey had a similar problem but with his sister."

"What happened to Jeffrey?" asked Suzanna.

"I haven't heard from my sister Lena for twelve years now. I contacted a search firm," said Jeffrey. "They gave me an address in Washington State. I wrote to her at that address, but the letter was returned with no forwarding address. I called the police where she had lived but they couldn't help me."

"Maybe she'd dead," said Gino. "It would explain everything."

"That's very sad, Jeffrey. I'm sorry this happened to you," said Suzanna very nicely.

"I hope she's not dead," said Paisley.

"Maybe she was murdered," said Mary. "She might be on one of those crime shows that they make so many of today."

"I don't think you should focus on the negative side," suggested Suzanna. "I think hopefully his sister Lena will contact him eventually. It could be a case of a simple misunderstanding."

"Don't give up hope Jeffrey," said Roberta. "I would leave it in the hands of the lord. He'll find her somehow."

"That's right," said Suzanna. "The next stressor is working with incompetent people. I don't have that problem. Everyone here at Campbell Care is very competent."

"I've had that problem," said Gino. "I keep on having that problem. I've quit jobs in the past because of that."

"I can imagine that's very frustrating," sympathized Suzanna, as she smoothed down her brown hair.

"The next stressor is 'not being able to find a Kleenex and needing it.' Major or minor?"

"Minor," said Gino.

"Birth of a child?" asked Suzanna.

"Major stressor," said Jessica. "I know from experience. Giving birth to my two sons was a joy and blessing but also hard as hell on my body. But I wouldn't trade it for anything."

"I agree with Jessica," said Mary. "My children are a blessing every day of my life."

"I don't have any children of own yet," said Roberta. "But I'm sure it will be a wonderful thing. I think my doctor told my husband that I can't have children."

"What about this one 'being late on a deadline'?"

"Yes, I can relate to that one," said Paisley. "I used to work as an editorial assistant at a small weekly trade journal in Washington, D.C. Our deadline was Friday. Some of the reporters would come just under the gun."

"That must have been very stressful, Paisley," said Suzanna.

"Yes, it was," said Paisley. "But it taught me how to write under stress better."

"The next one is 'Having In-law problems.'"

"My husband's parents adored me," said Mary. "They treated me like I was their own daughter."

"My in-laws and I got along well," said Jessica. "But I know other people who have problems with them like that old TV show 'The Mothers-in-Law.'"

Lois tilted her head a little and had a thoughtful look on her face. She looked as if she was going to talk. Liza yawned, finding this group very boring.

"Now this one 'problems at the boarding house'?" asked Suzanna.

"No, I get along okay," assured Annie. "But sometimes the food is lousy. I think that it could have too much sugar in it and I'm diabetic."

"Living at home with my mother can be as bad as living in a boarding home," said Liza. "Sometimes she really put the 'cunt' back into 'country.'" Gino and Paisley burst into laughter.

"Liza! Okay. 'Recent death of someone close to you.' Major or minor?" asked Suzanna.

"I was very upset when my mother died," said Paisley. "We had a month to clean out her apartment."

"I only had three weeks to clean out my mother's apartment," said Gino solemnly. "That was very stressful. I was the one who found her dead. She was lying in bed. My sisters paid for the funeral."

"I can imagine," said Paisley. "That must have been very hard."

"Tell me about it," said Gino sarcastically. "That's why I moved into Easter Seals. I couldn't afford to pay the rent on my own."

"Well, yes. I had a recent death of someone close to me," said Liza. "My grandmother, my mother's mother, died last year. She was my best friend."

"Do you have any brothers or sisters?" asked Suzanna.

"No, I don't," said Liza. "It was just me."

"Being an only child must be hard," said Paisley. "All of my friends who are only children wish they had a brother or sister."

"I tried to kill myself after my father died," said Mary. "I really loved him more than I ever did my mother."

"I wanted to kill myself after my mother died," said Annie. "But my aunt sends me money for my birthday every year. I have a brother, but I hate him. He's the devil."

"I'm glad that both of you were unsuccessful in your suicide attempts," said Suzanna. "It was not your time to leave this earth yet."

"You should leave that in the hands of the almighty," said Jessica. "Let him decide when you should go. It's his decision not ours."

"I know that now," said Mary. "It's a sin to kill yourself. I don't want my soul to end up in purgatory."

"Living in a boarding home is like being in purgatory," said Gino.

"Suicide is a permanent solution to a temporary problem," quoted Suzanna.

"It's also against the law to kill yourself," said Gino.

"That's a stupid law," said Liza. "How are going to arrest someone for killing themselves when they're already dead?"

"That's true," agreed Suzanna. "Think of all the people who would be upset if you killed yourself. Your friends, your parents and your husband. Your life touches so many other people's lives."

"I don't want to talk about death," said Lois. "Can we talk about something else? Like food, do you believe they can make synthetic food?"

"She was talking about that yesterday," said Gino impatiently. "Why does she talk about such bullshit?"

"I don't know about that Lois," said Suzanna. "But I'm unwilling to find out. The next stressor is 'Having difficulty motivating yourself.' Major or minor?"

"Major," said Mark. "Some days I don't want to get out of bed. I don't want to shave; I don't want to take a shower. But I come to Campbell Care anyway."

"I know what Mark means," said Jessica. "I don't like coming here every day. Some days my arthritis bothers me so much I don't want to get out of bed."

"I guess we all feel that way sometimes," said Mary. "Especially if I have a bad headache."

"I don't want to come here every day, but I come to program because I have nothing to do at home," said Annie. "I don't want to just lay around the house all day watching soap operas. That would be boring."

"I like coming here," said Lois. "This is like my second home. I enjoy coming to Campbell Care."

"I'm happy to hear that," said Suzanna. "We want everyone to like coming here. If you have suggestions on improving Campbell Care, drop them in the suggestion box in the APR. It's right near the assistant director Cynthia's office."

The bell rang as usual ending this period and signaling Paisley and others to go to the second lunch in the APR.

"You know what I consider the biggest stressor, Suzanna?" asked Annie. "Being in love with someone who doesn't love you. Have you ever that happen to you?"

"Yes, I know," agreed Suzanna. "That's really like being in purgatory."

Everybody left Room 9 to go to lunch, even though the lunch was never very special. Its main quality was that it was always free. Cooking lunch for more than one hundred people probably was the reason why the menu at Campbell Care had to be easy to prepare and cheap. It also was bland because many of the consumers there had diabetes or hypertension.

Chapter 11

Some of the groups at Campbell Care were not obviously therapeutic. They were mainly recreational. They had an underlining purpose of encouraging social intercourse amongst the patients who attended Campbell Care. People could choose the groups that they wanted with their counselors. These were the groups called hobbies games and cards, and bingo. Paisley had decided to be in the bingo group which was held every Friday after lunch in the APR.

Paisley lingered in the APR after lunch, which on Fridays was usually a fish sandwich or a little pizza with a salad. The salad was iceberg lettuce strips of carrots, strips of red cabbage, and chunks of tomatoes. This Friday they had the pizza, which you would get after waiting in line and going up to the window of the kitchen. Some people called the pizza "hockey pucks" because they were round and sometimes too hard to chew easily.

There were about five other people in the APR. There was Linda sitting at the receptionist desk talking on a land line telephone. John one of the security guards, who was also black like most of the support staff, sat at the security desk. There were three people still eating lunch seated at the brown collapsible tables in the APR.

At one o'clock Linda pressed the white button on the wall behind her next to the doorway of Cynthia's, the assistant director, office. That button controlled the buzzer which signaled throughout the entire building the beginning and ending of each period of group therapy.

About twenty people entered the APR and got bingo boards from the round table in the front of the APR. The table was in front of the white board whereupon Paisley wrote in erasable magic marker the current date. The board was between the doorway leading to the kitchen and a doorway leading to two bathrooms. Each bathroom was labeled "Women" or "Men." Some places wanted to have gender neutral bathrooms, but the staff figured that would encourage sexual activity in them.

"Okay," said Eddy. "Get your boards and chips and then we'll begin the games."

There were two counselors who ran bingo. Eddy and Jose, a handsome Latino who also ran the workshop. Paisley thought it was a little surprising that he had two children even though he was only twenty-six years old. Most of Paisley's relatives had waited until they were in their thirties before having any offspring.

"I'll bring around the sign in sheet," said Jose.

Every group had a sign in sheet. This proved to all the counselors that the patients in their home groups had actually attended the therapy groups to which they were assigned. Likewise, Medicaid wanted to have proof that patients where receiving the therapy which they were supposed to. Medicaid provided the major funding for the program. Some of it came from donations or private insurance companies. Most of the patients went to the program voluntarily, but some were sent there by court orders.

Paisley sat at the table next to the soda machine where he usually sat. Kenneth sat across from Paisley at the very end of the table in his favorite spot.

"Hi, Kenneth," said Paisley.

"Hi, dude. Did you get a board with 069 on it?"

"Of course, I did," answered Paisley sheepishly. "And I also had 070 because they always call that."

Paisley and Kenneth both knew the number 69 referred to a certain kind of sex act. For gay men it meant mutual fellatio between two men. He felt what you did at the same time, because your penis was in his mouth and his was in yours. Sometimes you experienced orgasms at the same time too.

The person who was calling the bingo numbers was Franklin, a 48-year-old African American man with a clean lucid voice. The numbers were on little red balls with white lettering in a large mesh metal globe that spun around.

On the front of the wooden round table were several bingo prizes. They were toiletries like soap, maxi pads, shampoo, toothpaste and cologne. Campbell Care wasn't allowed to offer cash prizes like other bingo games at some local churches in New Jersey. The authorities probably were worried that somebody would spend a cash prize on scratch-offs, alcohol or illegal drugs.

As usual not everyone won a bingo game. What was probably a relief to everyone was that Annie won a game. She got so excited that someone thought she was having an orgasm. Paisley never cared very much whether he won or not. Because of his family's occasional help, he usually had enough money to buy his own toiletries. When he won something at Bingo, he often gave it away to someone like Lois or Kenneth who could use it more than he did.

Mark, a native of Turkey with a large head approached the soda machine.

He placed a one-dollar bill in the designated slot. He pressed two buttons and a bottle of Pepsi fell to the bottom of the machine. He removed the plastic bottle and unscrewed the top with his left hand.

"Hi, Paisley. Hi, Kenneth."

"Hi, Mark."

"Did I tell you the great joke I heard once?" asked Mark.

"No, you didn't."

"It goes like this! Are you a smart fella, or are you a fart smellah?" Mark laughed at his own joke.

"Oh my God," said Mary in disgust. "You pig!"

"You're a piece of work, Mark," chuckled Annie. "I always love your jokes!"

"Why don't you two slobs get married?" said Mary. "You both think alike."

"Now that would be funny!" exclaimed Kenneth.

Because it was St. Patrick's Day, and also the third Friday of the month, the Bingo games were cut from a full hour to thirty minutes. There was a birthday party after Bingo, where people who had a birthday that month were seated at the same table from which Franklin called the bingo numbers. Likewise, the rest of the people at Campbell Care got cake and ice cream on little Styrofoam plates. There was diabetic cake and ice cream as well which Paisley and other diabetics consumed.

After the birthday party on the third Friday of each month, there was always a talent show. In the talent shows run by Eddy, people who had signed a list would sing along with CDs that they had chosen themselves. This program could not afford a karaoke machine. Eddy usually determined the order in which people performed by the attendance record of each person. Because he had been away for two weeks taking care of his brother and sister-in-law's dog Buddy, Paisley was the third to last to perform, due to his relatively bad attendance.

Nine people in all sang in the talent show this time. Three were men and six were women. Most of them sang the same songs that they always sang at the talent shows. Those were often ones that were popular in the 1970s and 1980s. One of the songs was almost always one sung originally by Whitney Houston. Paisley decided to sing a tune which came out in 1965 called "I'll Never Find Another You." It was made famous by a folk rock group called The Seekers who were from Down Under. They also sang the theme song to the movie Georgy Girl.

Paisley's favorite line in that song was "If I searched the whole world over until my life is through, I know I'd never find another you." Paisley used to think of his ex-lover Boris, whenever he had heard this song. Now he thought of the man whom he secretly loved, Jim, whenever he sang that song. He wanted to dedicate this beautiful song to him but didn't dare to for fear of embarrassing him.

Several people sang before Paisley. Lois did an off-key rendition of "The Girl from Ipanema." A black lady named Lydia sang a gospel song called "Wade in the Water."

Annie always cheered Lydia on because she was her best friend.

"That was great," said Eddy after Paisley finished singing 'Hitchin' a Ride' by Vanity Fare. "You have such cool taste in music."

Paisley walked back to the hard, plastic chair where he had sat during the bingo. Kenneth was still sitting in his same seat too. Jim was sitting on the other side of Paisley.

"Good job," said Jim, smiling at Paisley.

"That was a wonderful song," said Mary.

"Thank you," responded Paisley. "Did you recognize that song?"

"Yes, I did," said Jim. "It came out in the sixties when I was just a boy."

"My brother Plaid Jubilee was eight years old when it came out in 1968," said Paisley. "My other brother Argyle would have been thirteen years old, so he probably remembers it well."

"I would have been eight then too," said Jim. "Because I'm five years older than you and you were born in 1965. Right?"

"Yes, you're right," agreed Paisley "My favorite time period of music is from the 1960s and 1970s. I also like some jazz, because my parents played it a lot."

"I like that kind of music too," said Kenneth. "I also like the eighties. Hall and Oates, Tina Turner, Prince, Shaka Khan, David Bowie."

"Yeah, I love Led Zeppelin," said Jim. "And Pink Floyd, Rush, The Rolling Stones and Jethro Tull."

"I love the Beatles," said Paisley "The Rolling Stones, The Supremes and Blondie."

"I love Motown," said Kenneth. "And Abba."

"Everybody loves Abba," said Paisley. "I love Blondie and the B52's."

"The B52's?" asked Jim.

"Yes, the fact some of them are gay helps too," said Paisley. "They are very campy and amusing with their funny clothing."

At that time that they were talking, the last three people performed in the talent show. Then Eddy conducted his fashion show which he narrated by talking over the microphone, while five women walked around the APR. Most of them had help with their makeup Their funky clothes were from a local thrift store that Eddy liked called 'Second Hand Rose.'

Jim and Kenneth laughed at the same time Paisley said the word "gay."

"I didn't know that they were gay," said Kenneth.

"Yes, they said so in a Rolling Stone magazine interview. I think that they revealed that they were gay," explained Paisley. "I liked them before I knew about this anyway. It isn't always instrumental in my decision to like any group, but it can help me a little."

"That makes a lot of sense to me," said Jim. "It doesn't matter to me whether or not a music group is gay or not."

"Most of them are in the closet until someone or something outs them," said Paisley. "Like what happened in the case of George Michael."

"Right, I heard about that," said Jim. "It was in all the papers."

"Aren't there other celebrities who were rumored to be gay. Jodie Foster, Leonardo DiCaprio, Neil Patrick Harris," said Paisley.

"Oh yeah. I don't see why it matters so much to people," said Jim. "I don't care about that. I never have."

"I don't either," agreed Kenneth.

"I had trouble at my first college, St. John's College. I left there after just three semesters because of the harassment that I had to endure," said Paisley.

"I don't blame you if it was that bad," said Jim. "Teenagers are confused about their sexuality and treat others badly. They're very insecure about themselves."

"Being openly gay is very risky," said Kenneth very quietly. "You open yourself up for trouble. I've had more trouble from females than males, however. You should never admit that here."

"They were probably attracted to you and lashed out at you because they felt rejected by you," said Jim. "Women are trouble."

"Yes, you have a very good point. And then I've had some supposedly straight men ask if I want to give them a blow job," said Paisley. "And on some rare occasion I've had people who have come to me after I came out to them, including my cousin Jessica."

"Your cousin is gay, too?" asked Jim.

"Yes, my cousin is a lesbian," answered Paisley. "Her parents have had trouble dealing with one of their children being gay."

"I have four children," said Jim. "It wouldn't matter to me if any of them were gay. I would still love them anyway."

"You're a very unusual man, Jim," said Paisley. "But that has been obvious to me since I first met you. That's one of the reasons why I…like you so much."

"Thank you, Paisley."

"You not only have a nice face and good voice but also a beautiful soul," said Paisley.

"Thank you, I like you very much too. But in a platonic way not romantically."

At that moment the bell rang, signaling not only the end of the talent show but also the end of another day and week at Campbell Care.

Paisley, Jim, Kenneth and the rest of the patients headed toward the front door.

"Have a good weekend everybody," said Eddy. "Remember to stay away from people, places and things."

"Have a good weekend Jim," said Paisley.

"You too, Paisley," said Jim, patting him on the left shoulder.

Paisley felt an electric pulse pass through his body from Jim's touch.

"See you Monday," said Paisley.

"See you Monday," said Jim.

Paisley got into Gabby's van as he had many times before, feeling sentimental thinking about Jim's hand on his shoulder. Kenneth settled into the back seat in the right-hand corner of the van. He put on his black sunglasses. Mary got into the front seat, next to Gabby.

"Why are you sitting in the back seat, Kenneth?" joked Paisley. "Don't you remember what Rosa Parks did."

"I had an aunt named 'Rosa Parks,' dude."

"Do you really mean that?" asked Gabby their van driver from Puerto Rico.

"Yeah right," said Mary. "And I had an uncle named Sam!"

"Mary Christmas thinks you are joking, Kenneth," said Gabby in a silly tone of voice.

Franklin got into the van. Then they drove away from Campbell Care for another weekend.

Chapter 12

Among the many types of groups that were offered at Campbell Care, there was one which was very different from the others. It was called poetry therapy. This poetry group Paisley attended twice a week. The counselor who ran it was named Polly Sanchez. She would obtain poetry from the Internet in her office. The patients in this group would read the poems. She usually found four or five poems and then they would discuss them. Occasionally someone brought in a book of poetry from home from which to read.

Polly Sanchez was a thirty-two-year-old woman of Portuguese ancestry. She was married to a Spanish policeman. She had gotten back from her maternity leave about six months after giving birth to twin boys. Although she had lost all of her pregnancy weight, she was still self-conscious about her appearance.

"When I had a big belly, everyone ignored my big nose!" she said one day.

She had a pleasing face with big brown eyes and full lips, but her nose was a little bit too big for her face. It really was not noticeable when you saw her from the front. When she turned to look at something, then you could see what she meant. Her physical beauty may have been flawed but her personality was beautiful on its own merits. If there had been a beauty pageant for the female social worker with the most attractive personality, Polly would have won it easily.

Polly had worked at Campbell Care for eight years, longer than any other counselor. Therefore, she remembered all of the counselors who had come and gone from Campbell Care. Most of them were young women who had only worked there one or two years before leaving for another higher paying job. Polly's opinion was that the field of psychotherapy had always had a high turnover rate. Campbell Care was no exception to that rule.

As he usually did, Paisley got to Room 1, where poetry therapy always was held, before everyone else. Paisley had read that Virgos are like that. They are the first to arrive and the last to leave anywhere. His mother had seemed more concerned about the zodiac signs than most people. It had been a fad during the 1970s to ask other people the question "What sign are you?" Some people still asked Paisley that silly question. He only pretended to care about that sort of thing, merely to humor other people.

Paisley could see outside through a metal door at the far end of the room. It was partially open, and the sun shone into the room.

"Hi, Joy," said Paisley. "How are you?"

"I'm a little tired," said Joy, sitting down on one of the black plastic chairs with metal legs. "I had trouble sleeping last night."

Joy was a nice 55-year-old woman from Trinidad. Her parents were originally from India, so that Joy had a dark complexion. She had long black hair which she usually wore in a braided ponytail. However, she had a Trinidadian accent instead of an Indian one. She was one of the few Hindus whom Paisley knew socially.

"I take Seroquel for insomnia, Joy," explained Paisley. "I used to have nightmares."

As the bell rang, more people entered Room 1. Most of them sat down around a rectangular, brown collapsible table like the ones in the APR. Others sat in chairs that were arranged along the plain white walls. There was Mary, Mark, Annie, Lois, Gino, and Kenneth. After that Polly herself entered the room and sat down at the head of the table. She had a bunch of photocopies of poems and a legal notepad with a black ink pen.

"How is everybody today?" asked Polly. "Please sign in."

Polly handed a clipboard with a computer-generated list of names to Paisley. It was like the ones used in every therapy group. She passed out the copies of the poems. On the bottom of each page was written the web site where she had obtained the poetry and the date that she printed them out.

It was clear that most of these poems were not written by professional writers. Many of them had grammatical mistakes that were plainly obvious to a former proofreader like Paisley. Many of the poems did not rhyme. Paisley's taste in poetry was somewhat old fashioned in that he preferred poems that did rhyme.

"Who would like to read the first poem?" asked Polly cheerfully. "This group will be very long if I don't get any volunteers."

"I will," said Annie. "It's called 'When I see your Face.'"

"When I see your face,
I think of lovely things.
When I see your face,
I hear crystal springs.
When I see your face,
I see pretty tulips.
When I see your face,
I see your sweet two lips.
When I see your face,
I picture blues skies.
When I see your face,
I can see the sunrise.
When I see your face,
My life is complete.
By Jelly Donut."

Annie burst into laughter after she read the name "Jelly Donut."

"Jelly Donut?" asked Annie jokingly. "That name is even stranger than your name 'Paisley Jubilee'."

"Do you think you could get us some jelly donuts some day?" asked Gino hungrily. "I love those cream filled donuts too."

"Yes, I know I must," said Polly, winking at Paisley. "I'll bring a dozen assorted donuts next time we meet."

"Aren't you diabetic, Gino?" asked Joy, with concern.

"Yes, but I cheat sometimes," said Gino. "I can't help it. Maybe my bipolar disorder makes me eat too much?"

"From your big belly that's obvious," commented Mary. "I guess you could play Santa Claus."

"What do you call that?" asked Polly. "'Jelly Donut' can't be the real name."

"An alias?" said Mary. "That girl is definitely not a diabetic."

"It's a nom de plume," said Paisley triumphantly. "That means a pen name."

"Whatever," said Mary. "That's probably not his real name."

"Or *her* real name," said Polly. "Jelly Donut could be a man or a woman. It's a pseudonym. That's the word!"

"Maybe Jelly Donut works at Dunkin Donuts," said Paisley.

"What?" said Annie. "All this talking about donuts is making me very hungry."

"You're always hungry," said Mary. "That's sort of obvious."

"I like donuts too," said Lois. "And cupcakes, napoleons, éclairs, and peach cobbler."

"Okay, this isn't a baking class," said Polly "Let's move on to another subject besides fattening food. What does this poem mean to everyone?"

"I like the line where Jelly Donut says, 'I see pretty tulips, I see your sweet two lips,'" said Gino. "I wish I had a girl with two lips to kiss."

"That's very cute," said Polly. "I like it too."

"It's a pun," said Kenneth. "Two lips and 'Tulips."

"Okay yeah I was thinking of that too," said Paisley.

"Jelly Donut has a sweet way with words," said Mark. "I could use a donut right now myself. A Boston crème donut in fact."

"Oh my God!" said Mary. "Can we please stop talking about food?"

"I know," said Polly. "Let's move on to the next poem. Who would like to read it?"

"I will," said Mary.

"Your Super Duper Love.
You are my superman.
Your super-duper love makes me feel
Shiny and new like a beautiful rainbow.
Your super-duper love makes me feel
Soft and fuzzy inside like a cuddly teddy bear
Like nothing I've ever felt before.
Thank you, dear.

by Della Cox."

"What about this poem?" asked Polly. "Any thoughts on this one?"

"Della Cox?" said Kenneth. "What kind of name is that? That sounds like a porn star."

"My favorite porn star was Linda Lovelace," said Mark. "She was gorgeous and had big boobs."

"Paisley and Mark!" said Polly indignantly. "Really now. Keep it PG rated, please."

"My favorite part was about the beautiful rainbow," said Mary. "I love rainbows."

"Me too," said Joy. "I remember once seeing a double rainbow in Trinidad. It was a miracle from the Lord."

"I like rainbows too," said Polly. "Everybody does, I guess."

"I like the rainbow flag," said Paisley. "It's better than the pink triangle."

"What's the pink triangle?" asked Kenneth.

"The Germans made homosexuals wear them on their clothes in the concentration camps during World War II."

"Well now, let's go on to the next poem," said Polly. "Who wants to read this one?"

"Me," said Joy. "This one is called 'Your Face.'"

"Your face, a haggard wasteland,

Rains bitter tears on my harvest.

Like hungry locusts,

Your acidic words devastate my garden of compassion.

Your meanness pathetically rendered my life a vast desert.

And so I'll bid you goodbye.

I hope you die,

You miserable wretch.

by Alla Carte."

"Clearly this woman had serious issues," said Polly. "Who do you all think she's talking about? Her minister?"

"Her cousin," said Paisley. "I know from experience how awful they can be."

"No, I think it's her husband," said Mary. "She probably wrote this poem before she got a divorce from her abusive husband."

"I think so too," agreed Joy. "She says this to me with the words 'Your acidic words devastate my garden of compassion.' She is hurt by her husband's verbal abuse.

And I believe that his verbal abuse may have led to physical abuse. I feel this very strongly."

"I think you're probably right about this," said Polly. "Alla Carte seems to be a very troubled person. I can imagine her going through a lot of turmoil in her life."

"I think you're reading more into this than there is," said Mark. "I think that she is talking about herself. She's having her period."

"Whatever," said Polly, politely ignoring Mark's offensive remark. Her training taught her to avoid unpleasant comments by pretending not to hear them. Some mentally ill people had trouble censoring their impolite comments.

"Who wants to read the next poem?"

"I'll read it," said Kenneth. "I don't mind reading one of these priceless gems."

"069."

"Playing bingo, I never slumber.
Then I hear my favorite number.
When the bingo caller calls you
I feel fresh like summer dew.
I want to make love to you.
It's better than my wonderful weed.
Now I know I'll really succeed.
When I hear '069'
I'll feel really fine,
All of the time.
This is the end of my rhyme.

by John List."

"So, what does everyone think of this poem?" asked Polly. "Do you like it?"

"John List obviously likes playing bingo," said Mary. "I like playing bingo too even if I don't win anything."

"Are you in the bingo therapy group every Friday?" asked Polly.

"Yes, I am," said Mary. "It's one of my favorite groups beside this one."

"Thank you for that lovely compliment," said Polly. "Is anyone else in the bingo group?"

"Yes, I am," said Paisley "I love bingo. I like other games too like Scrabble, Yahtzee, and Sorry. I used to play them with my older brothers Argyle and Plaid."

"Do you still play those games?" asked Polly.

"Yes, of course I do. My friend Kenneth comes over once a month or so and plays Yahtzee and Scrabble with my roommate Jeffrey and me," said Paisley. "Kenneth is an excellent player. He often wins at Scrabble."

"I like Scrabble too," said Joy. "It keeps your mind active. So does knitting."

"I do those circle word finds too," said Annie. "They give you something to do at the laundromat waiting for your clothes to dry and also in the talking place."

The Talking Place was the name for Room 1A. If your group was canceled or you didn't feel well, you could go to the room called The Talking Place. However, every patient needed a permission note from the counselor who was running the group from which you wanted to be absent. Paisley would go there if Juan did not have any flours for him to pack. There was a large rose-colored sofa in there where many people took unauthorized naps.

"Do you ever play bingo, Kenneth?" asked Polly.

"No, but I used to like bridge," said Kenneth. "But not The Bridge over the River Kwai."

"I assume that John List likes bingo because of the poem he wrote," said Paisley. "I know how exciting it is to get really close to a bingo and need only one more number."

"Then the bingo caller calls your number. You shout out 'Bingo!' like that," said Annie. "It's almost like getting close to coming and them 'Pow'!"

"I never thought of it that way before," said Mark quizzically. "You've got a very good point. The tension builds up with each number called. Then you just read one more number and then 'Bingo' just like that. You almost want a cigarette after words."

Everyone laughed at Mark and Annie's very risqué comments except for Polly. Her mouth silently turned down at the corners.

"I don't know about that," said Joy, "I don't smoke anything if you know what I mean."

"I bet someday marijuana will be legal in California," predicted Mark.

"I quit smoking before I had my baby," said Polly, "although ever once in a while I get the craving for just one good drag on a cigarette. Let me feel the nicotine kick in. Then the impulse passes."

"All I ever smoked was reefers in my twenties," said Paisley. "And that was very rarely. My cousin Jessica liked to get me stoned. It was like a big game to her."

"Your cousin sound like a really charming person," said Polly. "Only kidding!"

"My brother Plaid is ten years older than me. He was an alcoholic, and my cousin Jessica has been smoking weed since she was thirteen," said Paisley. "I think they shouldn't need to self-medicate themselves."

"You're probably right," said Mary.

"I like to self-medicate with a jelly donut," said Gino. "Or a banana split."

"I think the years of smoking weed may have changed Jessica's whole personality," said Paisley woefully.

"Yes, I know," said Polly. "It sounds like she has been very paranoid."

"Marijuana smoking can change your personality," said Kenneth. "I've heard any drug abuse will mess up your mind. I know so because I've met people like that. Your cousin isn't that unusual. Loads of baby boomers have experimented with all kinds of drugs."

"So, we all agree that drugs are bad," said Polly. "Especially when taken with psychotropic medications like the ones that everyone at Campbell Care takes. You can have very bad side effects."

"Can it kill you?" asked Joy.

"I guess so," said Paisley hesitantly. "It probably could."

"Especially if you're using junk like heroin or ecstasy," said Joy. "Believe me, baby. I know people who did that stuff."

"Are you MICA, Joy?" asked Paisley.

"Yes, I am. So, I know what I'm talking about," said Joy wearily.

M.I.C.A. stands for mentally ill Chemical abusers. It refers to people who have a "dual diagnosis" of mental illness as well as illegal drugs or alcohol. The M.I.C.A. therapy groups at Campbell Care were tailored to this type of patient. Paisley's gay black friend Kenneth was also M.I.C.A., because he used to have a drinking problem. Some patients attended twelve step groups after program was over like Alcoholics Anonymous or Narcotics Anonymous.

"What's your drug of choice, Joy?" asked Paisley.

"That's a very personal question, Paisley," said Polly. "You don't have to answer that question if it embarrasses you, dear."

"I don't mind answering his questions," said Joy, "I've tried just about everything, Paisley. Weed, coke, booze, whatever. Sometimes I think it's a wonder that I'm even alive."

"I'm glad you're alive," said Annie. "You're a wonderful person, Joy. Like your name, it is a joy to know you."

"Thank you, Annie," replied Joy. "You're pretty wonderful yourself."

Annie got up out of her seat and walked over to Joy. She gave Joy a big hug.

"I think I'm going to cry," said Polly. "I can feel the love in the room."

"We're all like family here," said Joy. "Would you like to see a picture of my grandson?"

"Yes, I would," said Paisley as she passed it to him. "He's a really nice looking. How old is he?"

"He's four," said Joy proudly.

"He's very good looking. He'll be handsome when he grows up. Tall, dark and handsome," said Annie. "But he'll still be way too young for me."

Joy laughed.

"Anyway," said Polly, smiling. "Does anyone have anything else to say about this poem called '069' by John List?"

"Well, the number '069' may be a little suggestion," said Mark. "Does anyone here know why anyone?"

"Yes, I do," said Paisley. "In fact, I've tried sixty-nine several times."

"What does it mean?" asked Joy. "Maybe my English isn't so good."

Mary whispered something into Joy's ear and Joy laughed.

"You must be kidding," said Joy to Mary.

"No, I'm not," said Mary. "If you don't believe you probably could ask Paisley all about that after group is over."

"John List is a dirty old man," said Paisley.

"Yes, he is," said Mary. "Just like Mark."

"So, what is everyone doing this weekend?" asked Polly. "Gino?"

"I'm going to watch the game on TV," answered Gino. "I love watching my sports."

"I'm going to visit my grandkids," said Joy. "I babysit for them a lot."

"I'm going to work on my new novel," said Paisley.

"What is it about, Paisley?" asked Polly. "And please keep your answer PG rated."

"It's about my life in the mental health system," said Paisley. "It's about mental illness."

"That sounds very interesting," said Polly. "I'd like to read it someday."

"I'd be glad to have you read it and tell me what you think of it," said Paisley. "If I ever finish it."

"Of course, you'll finish it," said Kenneth.

"What are you doing this weekend Mark?" asked Polly.

"I don't know," said Mark. "I'll probably go downtown to Broad and Market Streets in Newark."

"What about you, Mary?" asked Polly.

"Saturday I'll go for a walk if it's nice," said Mary. "Listen to the radio on my favorite station. Sunday I usually go to church. When My brother and I were children, my father would drop us off at Sunday School."

"What kind of music do you like, Mary?" said Polly.

"Classical mainly," answered Mary. "And gospel music sometimes. And Protestant church hymns."

At that point in time, the bell rang as it always did at the end of a period.

"Have a good weekend everybody," said Polly cheerfully.

"TGIF!" said Annie joyfully.

Very softly after everyone else left the room, Polly said something to herself. "Thank God indeed. I would go crazy myself if I did not have a weekend to relax." She left the room and locked the door behind her.

Chapter 13

The longer that Paisley went to Campbell Care, the easier it was to adjust to it. After weekends ended and Monday arrived, he was more able to change his mindset from idleness to alertness. Many of the counselors were glad to have a patient there like Paisley, because he was intelligent and contributed helpfully to group discussions. His home group counselor, Eddy, wished that Paisley could work at Campbell Care in some capacity. After going there for a while, Paisley sometimes seriously thought about becoming a peer counselor. That job did not require a B.A. in psychology.

Paisley's counselor had enrolled him in a therapy group called Life Skills. The main purpose of this group was to discuss issues that dealt with patients' coping with the problems of daily living. Some patients were sicker than others and needed more help doing things like shopping, laundry and bathing themselves regularly.

This group was run by different counselors. Sometimes it was run by Nathan Goldberg, a thirty-five-year-old balding Jewish man with tortoise shell glasses. Other times Hakim Greenwood, a thirty-year-old dark-skinned man, oversaw the Life Skills group. Hakim was one of the part time counselors who worked at Campbell Care. He worked there while he pursued his M.S.W. at Rutgers University.

Paisley entered Room 2. It was a long rectangular room with many brown plastic and chrome-legged chairs lining the walls. He sat in one of the brown chairs next to a collapsible brown table like the ones in other rooms at Campbell Care. Because the tables were so similar, they must have been bought on sale from some manufacturer.

Other people came into the room and sat down. Liza, Mark, Mary, Joy, Annie, Lois and Franklin also entered the room. A 45-year-old woman, Lucille Trimble also joined the group. She was apparently Irish American from her graying red hair, and green eyes like the Emerald Isle itself. Then the facilitator Hakim himself came in and took a seat.

"Good morning, Hakim," said Lucille, flirtatiously. "You look nice today. I like that shirt."

Hakim was wearing a long-sleeved white shirt with daffodil yellow polka dots.

"Thank you, Lucille," said Hakim. "How are you?"

"Not so great. Today Sept 17th is the tenth anniversary of my mother's death," said Lucille. "I still miss her very much. All I have to remember her by is this ring."

Lucille showed everyone a beautiful gold ring. It looked like two ropes wrapped around each other. Clearly it was at least 14 carat gold.

"I know how you feel," said Paisley. "I was very upset when my mother died."

"I know," said Lucille. "You told me that you tried to kill yourself."

"You tried to kill yourself?" asked Hakim.

"Yes, I did," said Paisley. "I took an overdose of my diabetes pills. They took me to the emergency room. A nurse stuck a long, small tube down by left nostril."

"I know about that sort of thing," said Liza. "I worked as an EMT for many years, so I've seen everything. Like *everything* for real. The real blood, sweat, and tears."

"I'm glad you didn't die," said Annie. "I wanted to kill myself after my favorite aunt died five years ago. She used to send me money for my birthday every year."

"That would have been a tragedy," said Hakim. "I don't think your mother or favorite aunt would have wanted that either."

"You're probably right," said Paisley. "I've been on psyche medication ever since then."

"I have an exercise for us to do," said Hakim. "I'm going to give each of you a copy of something to fill out."

Franklin distributed copies of an article with the title of "Fly Away and Let Go." It had seven sentences to finish in a blank line under the incomplete sentence. Hakim gave everyone about ten minutes to fill out the form.

"Okay who wants to go first?" asked Hakim.

"Me," said Joy. "The nickname I was called that I hated is 'Doogla.'"

"What does 'doogla' mean?" asked Hakim.

"My mother was Indian from India and everyone thought that I was half black and half Indian because I had curly hair. So, they called me 'Doogla.'"

"Is that a racist word?" asked Paisley. "It sure sounds like one."

"Yes, it is. I'm not half black," said Joy, "I'm all Indian. I learned some Indian recipes from my mama."

"Yes, I guess that you look Indian," said Hakim. "Who is next? Anyone at all?"

"I hated being called Squirrel," said Gino.

"Why did they call you squirrel?" asked Hakim.

"Squirrels like nuts," said Gino. "I guess they all thought I was nuts. Nasty thing was that."

"The nickname I was called that I hated is 'Chris,'" said Franklin. "My middle name is Christopher. I also hated the nickname 'Frankie.' Like Frankie Avalon and Annette Funicello."

"I've heard of them," said Hakim. "Who were they?"

"They were actors and actresses in all those beach party movies in the 1960s," explained Paisley. "Like 'Beach Blanket Bingo' and 'Muscle Beach Party.'"

"I used to love those movies," said Annie. "I thought Frankie Avalon was cute. I used to look like Annette Funicello."

"I hated being called Lucy," said Lucille. "Like 'I Love Lucy.'"

"That's nothing compared to what they used to call me," said Mark. "They used to call me 'watermelon head' because I've always had a big head."

"What about you, Mary?" asked Hakim.

"The nicknames or name I was called that I hated is 'Red,'" said Mary. "Because I used to be a natural red head. I used to hate having red hair, but now I love my gray and red hair. I also used to be called 'Pippie Longstockings' because of my red hair. I hated that."

"I'll go next," said Hakim, "I used to be called 'Blackie,' because I am so dark-skinned."

"Do you have any children?" asked Paisley.

"Yes, I have a son," said Hakim. "He's two years old."

"Is he as dark as you?" asked Joy.

"No, he isn't," said Hakim. "But he's still chocolate."

"He can't pass the paper bag test," said Kenneth.

"What the hell is that?" asked Annie.

"If your skin color is lighter than the color of a paper bag, you could probably pass as white," explained Kenneth. "I would not pass that test myself."

"What about you Paisley?"

"With a name like 'Paisley Jubilee' you must have been tortured to death," said Kenneth.

"Oh please," said Paisley. "I was called 'Ju Ju' like juju beads. I was called 'P.J.' too. I hated that. I sometimes thought of getting my name legally changed. But now I like my name. Nobody will forget me as long as they live."

"That's true," said Hakim. "I have never met anyone with your name before."

"The part of my body I hate the most is…"

"My stomach," said Joy. "I'm too fat."

"I hate my big feet," said Franklin.

"I like men with big feet," said Annie lewdly.

"I hate my feet too," said Lucille. "I have feet that are too big for a woman. I have masculine looking feet. My mother had beautiful feet."

"The part of my body I hate the most is my flabby stomach," said Paisley. "I really need to lose some weight."

"The part of my body I hate the most is my legs," said Mary. "I think I have scrawny legs like a chicken."

"I hate my head," said Mark. "People have always said that I have a big head."

"I hate my nose," said Gino. "You could ski off of my nose."

Several people laughed out loud.

"The part of my body I hated the most is…my flat feet," said Hakim. "I have trouble finding comfortable shoes."

"What about the next one 'My teachers always complained about my'…?"

"They complained about my voice," said Franklin. "I always sat in the back of the class and my teachers couldn't hear me very well."

"My teachers never complained about me," said Joy. "I never went beyond the sixth grade in Trinidad."

"My teachers always complained about me passing notes in class," said Mary. "Particularly with girlfriends about the cutest boys in class."

"They complained about me talking too much," said Lucille. "They said I was a chatterbox."

"My teachers complained about my handwriting," said Mark. "It was…what is that word?"

"Illegible," said Paisley.

"It was illegible," said Mark. "It still is pretty bad."

"You can write on computers now," suggested Hakim.

"My teachers always complained about my daydreaming," said Paisley. "I sometimes didn't pay attention in class. I was thinking of stories in my head. I've always wanted to be a writer. I think that God makes me want to write."

"My teachers always complained about my…bad handwriting," said Hakim. "Like Mark's teachers, I had illegible handwriting. Okay, let's move onto the next one. 'The mistake I've made that still bothers me is…'"

"Getting a divorce," said Lucille. "I never stopped loving Lloyd Trimble. But he cheated on me and so I divorced him."

"It's the opposite for me," said Paisley. "Getting married to my bisexual friend was a mistake. Thank God for divorce."

"You should have married me instead," said Liza. "I sometimes think if I got married to a man and pretended to be straight, my mother would get off my case."

Gino and Lucille giggled freely.

"One mistake I've made that still really bothers me is…"

"Not having more children," said Joy. "I wanted a big family, but my husband only wants to have two children."

"My biggest mistake was trying drugs," said Liza. "My life would have been a hell of a lot better if I had never been introduced to drugs, especially heroin."

"My biggest mistake," said Mark "Was dropping out of school. I am going to get my G.E.D. soon."

"My biggest mistake was cheating on my girlfriend," said Franklin. "I'd probably be married to her if I hadn't done such a stupid thing."

"Nobody's perfect," said Joy. "No human being is perfect. Only God."

"You can't spend the rest of your life beating yourself about your mistakes," said Hakim. "Try to learn from them."

Everyone stopped talking. Paisley sipped from his bottle of diet soda.

"I guess my biggest mistake was not going to college," said Gino. "I got sick and started hearing voices when I was getting ready to go to college."

"That's not your fault," said Joy. "You didn't get sick on purpose. Nobody asks God to make them sick in the head."

"That's true," said Hakim. "Nobody chooses to be mental ill. It's probably a chemical imbalance in your brain."

"I think mental illness is hereditary and possibly even genetic," said Paisley. "My mother and my cousin Jessica had been hospitalized for depression."

"I've heard of that too," said Mary. "I think I watched a special on that on the Discovery Channel. They said the same thing."

"I love that channel too," said Paisley. "I also love the Turner Classic Movies channel. I have recorded a lot of movies from that channel. My favorite movie is 'Casablanca' with Humphrey Bogart and Ingrid Bergman."

"I watched 'Forensic Files' on cable," said Liza. "It's fascinating to see how forensic science can solve what are supposedly perfect crimes. One lesbian was murdered by her married female lover and the lover's jealous husband."

"What!" exclaimed Mary. "You must be kidding, girl."

Liza and Paisley looked at each other. They chuckled together.

"Yes, I watch those too. There is no perfect crime," said Hakim. "What about the next one 'The negative thing I say to myself most often is…'?"

"I'm fat," said Paisley. "That's what I say to myself."

"I think I'm fat too," said Lucille. "Especially my thunder thighs."

"I don't think so," said Mark. "You're perfect to me. You have a nice face and nice big boobs."

"Yeah you are a cutie," said Liza.

"I don't allow myself to think negative things about myself," said Joy. "I concentrate on positive affirmations. I think of myself as a good person."

"I think that I am too fat too," said Mary.

"The negative thing I say to myself most often is 'I have a big head,'" said Mark.

"I sometimes think to myself that I am crazy," said Gino.

"I don't think, you're crazy," said Mary. "You shouldn't think of yourself that way."

"I don't feel anything negative about myself," said Franklin. "I like myself just the way I am."

"I agree with that too," said Hakim. "I don't try to emphasize bad things in my life. I need to be strong for my son."

"Neither do I," said Joy. "It'll make me go crazy and have another nervous breakdown."

"Here is the next one," said Hakim. "The thing that upsets me the most about other people is when they…?"

"Lie a lot," said Joy. "I hate it when people lie to me. I think that's a sin."

"I feel the same way," said Mary. "I always tell my brother not to lie, that honesty is the best policy."

"I agree with you on that," said Mark. "I want people to be honest with me. I hate girls who lie to me. It makes me mad."

"I hate it when people talk about me behind my back," said Lucille. "Back stabbers are such lousy bitches."

"Oh yeah," said Liza. "My girlfriend lied to me about leaving her husband."

"The thing that upsets me the most about other people is when they…"

"Eat with their mouth open. This is so disgusting!" said Mary. "And picking their nose."

Paisley made a smacking sound with his mouth.

"I hate it when people pretend," said Gino. "When they are making believe."

"You mean when they pretend to like you?" asked Paisley. "Is that it?"

"Yes, that's part of it," answered Gino. "Phony baloney people."

"You mean phonies?" asked Lucille. "I hate women who pretend to be my friend and then flirt with my boyfriend when I am not around. I could scratch their eyes out."

"I hate people who judge me," said Franklin. "I don't like being told what to do like their playing God. I hate when they call me 'stupid' too."

"I know what you mean," said Hakim. "I don't like people who are hypocrites. They pretend to be one thing and then do something else."

"Exactly, like I said phonies," said Lucille.

"Smiling faces, smiling faces sometimes they don't tell the truth," sang Franklin.

Everyone laughed. They probably recognized that Motown song from the decade of the 1960s. Paisley's older brothers always told him that the 1960s was the best time for rock and R&B music.

"The final one is 'The one thing that I always kick myself for is'…?" asked Hakim.

"Forgetfulness," said Paisley. "Sometimes I leave water boiling on the stove. Or I forget to lock my front door."

"You're having a 'senior moment,'" said Liza. "My mother does too."

"I guess my negative trait is smoking," said Kenneth. "I wish I could quit."

"I know," said Franklin. "I wish that I could quit too. But it's so hard."

"Cigarettes are so expensive now," said Lucille. "I can't afford them anymore, so I made myself quit. Besides they would make my clothes and breath smell bad too, like an ashtray."

"How much are they now?" asked Hakim.

"I hear they're seven dollars a pack now in New York City," said Lucille. "They're about six dollars a pack now in New Jersey. It's highway robbery. So are the loosies that stores sell to you one cigarette at a time."

"Getting high is highway robbery too," said Liza.

Everyone laughed at Liza's little pun. Liza's masculine appearance and sarcasm upset everyone at first. Her jokes made her seem nicer and more approachable after knowing her for a while.

"I quit smoking a year ago," said Mark. "The one thing that I have that I always kick myself for is procrastination. I wish I had gotten my G.E.D. ages ago."

"Better late than never," said Paisley. "You can't keep on beating up on yourself for things that you didn't do in the past."

"He's right," said Hakim. "It's good that you're doing something about this now instead of never."

"It doesn't matter the mistakes you made in the past," said Joy. "It's what you do now that matters. Just don't repeat history and meet your own Waterloo."

"The only thing that matters is that you always use a condom," said Mark. "Or that she is really on the birth control pill."

"Oh God!" said Mary. "Don't even get me started on STDs."

"I never sleep with men," said Liza. "So, I never need pills or an abortion."

Just then another therapy group ended as the buzzer went off in the entire building.

"We can continue this discussion next week," said Hakim. "Good work everybody!"

Chapter 14

Paisley did not attend very many therapy groups that were run by his own counselor, Eddy Aiken. Eddy led many of the therapy groups designed for the patients who were considered M.I.C.A. Paisley was not considered to be M.I.C.A. which was an acronym for Mentally Ill Chemical Abuser. The chemical dependency could be either illegal street drugs or alcohol. It was also deemed a "dual diagnosis," because the person involved had two problems, instead of just being mentally ill. All of the other patients in Eddy's home group were M.I.C.A. besides Paisley.

There was one group which Eddy led that Paisley attended called Coping with Loss. It was one of the few groups on Eddy's schedule which was not M.I.C.A. As the named implied, it was intended to help patients recover from a loss of any kind. Not necessarily a death, but it could be that as well as something such as the loss of a job or loss of a home. Many mental patients had been homeless at one time or another, sometimes as teenagers whose parents rejected them.

Coping with loss was always held in Room 4. Room 4 was different from the other rooms in that it was a large square room and was painted yellow like eggnog. It was lined with a bunch of mismatched chairs, all plastic with chrome legs. Room 4 had a ceiling which was higher than the other rooms. It also had no windows in it, like many of the other rooms at Campbell Care. Unlike most of Campbell Care, Room Four had a floor painted gray instead of blue and white tiling as in the APR.

As was frequently true, Paisley was the first person to enter the room. He sat in his usual corner. He pulled a bottle of diet cherry coke out of his well-worn Prado Museum. Canvas tote bag Its original beige color was now blotchy on the bottom of the tote bag from frequent use. He also kept a book of word finds, a pen, a copy of his weekly schedule, and a little notebook. He used the notebook to record ideas inspired by comments that people said during the day at Campbell Care. He thought of using these ideas to write a short story.

"Hi, Paisley," said Lucille. "How are you?"

Her emerald eyes were shiny over her lips, a perfect shade of red lipstick.

"I'm okay," said Paisley. "I can't wait until the weekend. How are you?"

"I'm fine, thank you," said Lucille sitting down.

Several other people entered the room: Joy, Deanna, Roberta, Jim, Mary, and Franklin. Joy was one of the few women at Campbell Care who usually wore dresses. Most of the female patients at Campbell Care wore pants or sweatpants at program. It could be that they could simply not afford anything else. Perhaps women from Trinidad like Joy dressed more conventionally feminine.

Eddy walked into the room wearing black pants and a dark green silk shirt. Paisley always thought that he was the coolest of counselors at Campbell Care. He always dressed better than most of the staff there, who often preferred to wear blue jeans instead of dress pants like his chinos or khakis.

"Hi, everybody," said Eddy as he sat in the chair nearest to the door. "I hope everyone is doing okay today. I know that I am."

"Hi, Eddy," said Joy. "You look good today."

"Hi, Joy. Thank you, dear."

Joy said exactly what Paisley was thinking too. Joy was one of a few ladies who were infatuated with Eddy.

"Thank you. How is everybody today?" asked Eddy.

"I'm okay," said Lucille. "I'm lucky to be alive."

"Just okay?" inquired Eddy. "That doesn't sound so good."

"It's near the anniversary of my sister Linda's death," said Lucille.

"You're having what's called an 'Anniversary Reaction,' Lucille. That's not so unusual around the time of something traumatic," said Eddy. "Like a divorce, getting fired or a death in the family. Coping with loss can mean the loss of anything. It could be the loss of your pet canary."

"She was only forty-one when she died. That's too young for anyone to die," said Lucille, very sadly.

"Yes, forty-one isn't that old," said Joy. "It's hard when you lose a sister. Particularly if she is younger than you. You are supposed to die first."

"I've been through hard times before," said Lucille. "My mother was born in the Great Depression. She remembered the long lines and ration stamps."

"That must have been a pain in the ass," said Paisley.

"They had to have no lights on and pull down the shades," said Lucille. "And then in World War II they had air raids and people put stars in their windows for each of their sons who had died. Now I think I know how they must have felt."

"That war was horrible for everybody," said Joy. "All wars are Hell."

"Hatred hurts the world," said Lucille.

"God hates war," said Deanna. "War is from the devil. And so are hateful people."

"Is anyone else feeling any kind of loss?" asked Eddy. "That is of course what this group is all about."

The entire group stopped talking. Some of the patients looked around the room as if they were trying to see who would speak next.

"Yes, I do," said Mary. "My mother died around this time. Even though she used to beat me, I still loved her."

"Your parents used to beat you?" asked Eddy.

"Spare the rod and spoil the child," said Joy. "Although I always heard that phrase, I rarely spanked my own children any way."

"Yes, my mother did," said Mary. "For no reason she used to beat me. She rarely touched my mentally challenged brother."

"Your brother was retarded?" asked Franklin.

"Yes, but I don't like that word," said Mary indignantly. "I consider it an insult to my brother."

"I'm sorry," said Franklin. "So your brother was slow?"

"I used to take care of my brother when my mother was in the hospital," explained Mary. "That's because my father was at work all day. I was like a second mother to him."

"What kind of a hospital was it?" asked Eddy.

"It was a mental hospital," explained Mary. "I think it was Greystone."

Greystone hospital was a mental hospital in New Jersey. It was a large, and old hospital where several of the patients at Campbell Care had been committed for months and even years in some cases. Paisley had never been a patient at that hospital. His friend Jim at this program had been there. Many politicians thought it was outdated and needed to be demolished someday.

"My mother was diagnosed as a paranoid schizophrenic," said Mary. "She was in University Hospital a few times when I was a girl."

"So, your mother was mentally Ill?" asked Paisley.

"Yes, she was," said Mary. "My father Ralph probably never should have married her in the first place. He said she seemed more normal when he first married her though."

"My mother was mentally ill too," said Paisley. "She also had major depression like me. That's one reason why I think that mental illness is hereditary, just like blue eyes or black wavy hair."

"Yes, it does seem to run in families, just like blue eyes or blond hair," said Eddy. "I've seen that before. More often than I would like to admit to anyone in fact."

"I think my mother was hearing voices that made her hurt me," said Mary quite sincerely. "My father was always good to me though. I feel sad visiting him now at the nursing home. Even though she's dead now, my father sometimes thinks I'm my mother. He asks me if he can leave with me."

"I wasn't aware you have had trouble with both parents," said Eddy. "Your mother you lost in reality. Your father you've lost in a way because his mind is slipping away from you."

"I know how hard it is to lose a parent," said Paisley. "My father deteriorated slowly because of his Parkinson's. I watched as his brain got worse and worse little by little and then he died."

"That must have been very difficult to live through," said Franklin.

"Have you had a loss of any kind Franklin?" asked Eddy.

"Yes, my girlfriend Lonnie died in May the 26th three years ago. My father also died a while ago," added Franklin. "I don't remember what day though."

"When that date comes up," said Eddy. "You might be feeling sad then?"

"I still mourn that loss," said Franklin, rubbing his eyes. "I was thinking about her when I had a car accident on the way to the cemetery to visit my father. My father was cremated but Lonnie was buried in a casket."

"The end of a relationship can be incredibly hard," said Eddy, sympathetically. "There's not only the guilt from losing someone important in your life but also the pain of seeing your hopes of a future life together disappear as well."

"I know exactly how you feel," said Lucille, "I still miss my sister. She was so young when she died. I feel funny being the survivor."

"That must have been tenable," said Paisley, looking at Franklin.

"It was," said Lucille. "Really awful."

"I met Lonnie in Overbrook," said Franklin.

Overbrook was the name for another mental hospital in Essex County in New Jersey. It was somewhat old like Greystone. It was located in Cedar Grove, New Jersey away from everything.

"We were together for eighteen years," added Franklin. "She died from lung cancer and pneumonia. I know that domestic violence is wrong. But I felt like it. Lonnie once stuck a knife in the doorway."

"She stuck a knife in the doorway?" asked Eddy. "Was she threatening you?"

"She had big arms," said Franklin. "When you get older you get bigger. She said if I cheated on her she would kill me."

"So, she did threaten you," said Eddy. "Women can cause domestic violence too."

"Hell hath no fury like a woman scorned," said Deanna. "God knows that's true."

"She got me bamboozled. But I didn't feel good when Lonnie died," continued Franklin. "I moved into a boarding home. I felt like drinking again. I got ill again. Psychotic. So, I was sent back to Overbook."

"You had something like a nervous breakdown," said Paisley. "The loss of Lonnie on top of your father's death made you sick again."

"I don't know if you could call it a 'nervous breakdown,'" said Franklin. "But I guess I did decompensate some."

"You have to realize that you're going to have to readjust how you see your future," said Eddy. "You are scared by the idea of having a life without Lonnie. But remember that in time you will get through this."

"It's hard to be alone," said Lucille. "I still miss my boyfriend Fred even though he has been dead for nearly five years. I'm just glad that he died before my sister did."

"Why is that?" asked Paisley.

"It would have broken his heart to see me lose her," said Lucille. "It would have killed him without the heart attack. I know it would."

"You're probably right about that," agreed Paisley. "That's the only benefit of it happening that way I guess."

"I still miss my mother," said Roberta. "Even though it's been four years, a day doesn't go by that I don't think about her."

"You must have been very close to her," said Jim.

"Yes, I was," said Roberta. "She was my best friend. If it wasn't for my husband Owen I don't know how I would have gotten through it."

"I didn't know that you were married," said Lucille. "How long have you been married?"

"Thirteen years," replied Roberta.

"Do you have any children?" asked Jim.

"No, we don't," said Roberta. "I don't know why."

"Is it possible that you didn't want children, or you just couldn't have any?" asked Paisley.

"We can't have any I guess," said Roberta. "But we use condoms and birth control pills any way for protection."

"Having no children doesn't always mean anything," said Paisley. "Jim has four children, and they almost never contact him."

"That's a sin," stated Deanna firmly. "God wants children to respect their parents."

"I don't understand how they can neglect him like that," said Paisley solemnly.

"A lot of mentally ill people are estranged from their families," said Eddy. "It often comes with the territory unfortunately. People are afraid of things that they don't understand."

"I know, but Jim is such a wonderful man that I find it hard to understand anyone treating him like this," said Paisley. "They don't know how lucky they are to have a father like Jim."

"It's okay, Paisley," said Jim. "I can handle it. Thanks for the compliments."

"Hearing that makes me sad," said Roberta. "If Jim was my father, I would do anything to stay in touch with him."

"Jim's situation is not that unusual," said Mr. Aiken.

"I often feel that my friends are more like my family than my actual family is," said Paisley. "This was true even before I became seriously ill."

"That's exactly right," said Eddy. "You can choose your friends, but you can't choose your relatives."

"Sometimes the staff at Easter Seals where I live treats me more like my family then my real family," said Paisley.

"I know what you mean," said Mary. "The staff at Project Live are like family to me. They're always nice to me."

Project Live was another residential program for mentally ill people like the one at Easter Seals. Paisley's friend Kenneth also lived at a Project Live house as Mary did. There were some options for housing besides the boarding homes. Project Live and Easter Seals did not take as much of their residents' social security checks as the boarding homes did. There were also some low-income housing projects run by the state of New Jersey as well, although these were sometimes in bad neighborhoods.

"I feel like the staff at Campbell Care is my family," said Roberta. "And so are my friends here too like Paisley and Jim. All this talk about family is making me sad. I need a hug."

Roberta got up from her chair next to Paisley and walked across Room 4 to where Eddy was sitting. Eddy rose from his chair and hugged Roberta. Lucille clapped.

"I need a hug too," said Paisley. "Would you give me a hug Jim?"

Jim stood up and hugged Paisley. Paisley felt so secure and safe in Jim's arms. Although he wanted to kiss him too, Paisley would never dare to actually do that. Normally everyone was discouraged from having any physical contact with each other.

Some patients were discharged for having sex in the bathrooms. That was probably the worst offense anyone could make, besides hitting a staff person. The security guards were intended to monitor any bad behavior there.

"This is all very touching," said Eddy. "Now let's get back to our discussion."

"What does it mean when you dream about someone who is now dead?" asked Paisley. "I dream about my father sometimes."

"I dream about my mother," said Roberta. "I still miss her very much. My dreams about her seem so real that it's scary to me."

"That's probably a desire to return to the past when everything seemed more secure and comfortable," said

Eddy very carefully. "You were feeling protected then when you were a child. Your parents took care of you. They took care of your housing, your food, your clothing. Everything that the boarding homes do now your parents used to do, and you felt happy and secure. You were longing for the past when your mother was alive. I dream about my father who died too."

"I have had a reoccurring dream about my dead friends and relatives," said Lucille. "In this dream I open a double door and in a big room are all my friends and relatives who have passed away. They are having a surprise party for me."

"Again, it's probably a desire to return to a time when you felt happier and more secure," said Eddy. "I could look this up in my dream book that I brought at Barnes and Noble. It explains what dreams about certain things mean. We can look at it during home group."

Home group was a period in the morning before all the other groups that each patient attended during the day. It was a time when each patient was with his or her counselor. Each counselor had about a dozen patients or so on his or her case load. Then there was a second home group before everyone left at 3:15 pm from Campbell Care. Paisley's home group was in a big room called Room 11. There were twelve full time counselors at Campbell Care, including Mr. Aiken, and each one had his or her own Home Group.

"I would like that very much," said Paisley. "I have had another recurring dream that I don't understand. I've dreamed that I was black."

"That's interesting," said Eddy. "Have you ever wished that you were black?"

"I'm not sure about that," said Lucille.

"Have you ever dreamed that you were white? Deanna?" asked Eddy, who was half black and half Asian. His eyes were Asian looking but his complexion was like café au lait.

"No, I haven't. That's stupid," said Deanna. "I'm proud to be black."

"Have you ever dreamed that you were white Roberta?" asked Eddy.

"Yes, I have," said Roberta. "One of my grandmothers was white."

"That's probably why she is light skinned," said Lucille. "A lot of black people have white ancestors in America, don't they?"

"You're probably right," agreed Paisley. "Could we look that up in your dream book?"

"Yes, we could," said Eddy, narrowing his eyes. "Definitely."

Paisley wondered if other white people have dreamed that they were black and if black people have ever dreamed that they were white. His thoughts were interrupted by the usual buzzer to signal the end of a therapy group. Paisley got up to go to the Happy Pharmacy across the street from Campbell Care. He often got cans of diet cherry coke, which they ordered especially for him.

Occasionally Jim would accompany Paisley. He would buy for himself a pack of Marlboro cigarettes. Unlike some smokers, however, Jim could make one pack of cigarettes last longer than a week. He was not as heavy a smoker as Kenneth. They still would please Paisley if they both could put aside tobacco forever.

Chapter 15

Over the few years that he had been going to Campbell Care, there were several groups that Paisley never attended, but that his friend Kenneth sometimes did. They were therapy groups for patients who were considered what is called M.I.C.A. These groups were called: M.I.C.A. Social; Staying clean; A.C.O.A.; contemplate sobriety; Anger Management; 12 steps; and spiritual Recovery.

One group however that Paisley did attend was one called "Social Group." It was supposed to help patients at Campbell Care learn about social interactions with other people. These social interactions could be anything from job interviews to dealing with a psychiatrist at a controlled environment like a mental hospital. Most of the patients had dealt with the former and all of them had dealt with the latter, including Paisley himself. However, he rarely ever discussed with his normal friends, who were *not* mentally ill, what it was like to be in a psychiatric ward.

Social group was usually held in Room 5. That room was comparatively small and painted lavender, while most of the other rooms at Campbell Care were painted an antiseptic shade of white. Social Group was run by an African American counselor named Steven Cornelius. He was originally from the Virgin Islands and had a slight accent.

Paisley entered the room and sat in his favorite purple chair, which was the only chair in Room 5 with arms. Behind this chair was a wall with a little window which investigated the staff lounge. On the other side of the window were white curtains that obstructed the view into the staff lounge.

Paisley had never been the only person in any therapy group. Sometimes his groups were cancelled when most of the assigned consumers were absent that day. Also, if the staff was shorthanded because one of the counselors was absent, a group would be cancelled.

Many patients at Campbell Care suspected that absent employees were out on job interviews. Eddy told him once in confidence that several counselors would leave Campbell Care because of the supposedly low salaries there.

Other people entered the room: Liza, Mark, Roberta, Joy, Lois, Alex, and Priscilla. Priscilla was a pretty forty-year-old black woman, who was always very friendly toward Paisley. She often dressed nicely, and some people thought she was a staff person there. Alex was a skinny middle-aged white man who smoked too much. His clothes sometimes smelt of tobacco smoke.

A few minutes later the counselor Steven Cornelius came into Room 5 and sat down next to the door, which was painted white like the other doors in Campbell Care. For privacy he shut the door behind him.

"How is everybody?" asked Steven.

"Okay I guess," said Liza. "I am here so I am alive."

"I was thinking of a question to ask you all," said Steven. "Then I'd like to see how you respond to it and how you react to strangers."

"I once took a ride from a guy in Florida," said Alex.

"What happened?" asked Steven.

"He turned out to be a homosexual," said Alex. "I got out of the car as soon as possible. He picked me up and then he tried to pick me up."

Liza and Paisley looked at each other and laughed. Over the last two years they had become good friends. Even though they were told not to discuss things at program, they would talk on the telephone about people at Campbell Care Liza's mother Anne asked her daughter Liza why she laughed so much, whenever Paisley called on her on her cell phone.

"Maybe you could have gotten a free blow job out of him," said Mark, half-jokingly.

"I didn't want to hang around long enough to find out," explained Alex. "I met some fruit loops in jail."

"Would you take a ride to Florida with someone that you just met?" asked Steven, looking at Roberta.

"No, I wouldn't," said Roberta. "He might try to attack me or something."

"What if it was a woman?" asked Steven.

"No, I still wouldn't trust her," said Roberta. "I wouldn't go anywhere with a stranger. I would have to know the person first."

"You could get to know him while driving on the trip down to Florida," said Steven.

"I would want to know the person before going on a trip somewhere," said Roberta emphatically. "Then I'd know that I could trust him."

"Trust is an important part of any relationship," said Paisley. "I like for instance let's say I'm on a job interview. The interviewer has to trust that I did not lie on my resume just to make me seem better than I am. It's hard to trust someone who is a stranger."

"You have to take risks in order to meet someone," said Steven. "Everyone that you know now was a stranger at one time. When you first got to Campbell Care everyone was a stranger to you."

"Not everyone," said Alex. "Some of the people here I knew before coming here. I met some of them at Greystone when I was there."

"Well, excluding that everyone here was a stranger when you first got here," said Steven.

"That's true," agreed Paisley. "Everyone including you."

"How did you get to know people here?" asked Steven. "You had to take risks to break the ice. What can you say to someone?"

"You can talk about the weather," said Priscilla. "That's always a safe subject that won't offend anyone."

"You can meet people anywhere," said Paisley. "My father and stepmother met through a personal ad in New York Magazine."

"You got to be kidding!" said Liza. "That is so weird."

"Would you be willing to meet someone through a personal ad, Alex?" asked Steven.

"No, I wouldn't," said Alex. "Only losers and hookers read personal ads."

"Would you Priscilla?" asked Steven.

"No," said Priscilla. "I also don't know if I would want to meet anyone over the internet either."

"How about you Roberta?" asked Steven.

"No," said Roberta. "Never in a million years."

"Mark?" asked Steven.

"I don't know," said Mark. "If her ad had a photo with it, maybe I would. Especially if she had nice tits."

"Would you Lois?" asked Steven. "Would you meet someone through a personal ad."

"No, I wouldn't," said Lois. "Only weirdoes, perverts, and con artists place personal ads in the newspaper."

"Would you answer a personal ad, Liza?" asked Paisley.

"I don't know," said Liza. "I agree with Mark, only if she had nice tits."

"Oh God!" said Mark. "Are you a lesbian?"

"Are you the alternative?" asked Liza.

"I always guessed you were gay," said Priscilla. "If you don't mind me saying so."

"No, I don't mind that," said Liza. "No offense is taken. I know I look kind of obvious to most people. I do it on purpose I guess."

"So almost no one would answer a personal ad Paisley," concluded Steven. "We've established that much so far. How do you meet other people then?"

"I met my first husband at the high school prom," said Roberta. "We dated for a while and then got married in a church."

"Would you even get married again?" asked Steve.

"No," said Priscilla. "Twice is enough for me."

"Once was enough for me," said Paisley.

"Were you married to a man or a woman?" asked Mark. "In my country Turkey gay men can't marry each other."

"To a woman," answered Paisley. "She was a former friend of mine whom I knew for 18 years."

"I thought you were gay," said Priscilla quizzically.

"My wife was a bisexual friend of mine whom I married because I was homeless," explained Paisley. "I got a no-fault divorce 18 months later that my ex-lover paid for."

"That was very nice of him," said Alex. "And it is also a little strange that your ex-lover paid for your divorce from your ex-wife."

"Yes, it was," said Paisley. "Otherwise, I would have to wait until I got my $8,000 retroactive payment from Social Security."

"Eight thousand dollars is a lot of money," said Steven.

"Yes, it is," said Paisley. "I've spent all of it by now. I bought a computer and a printer. I got a lot of new clothes that don't fit me anymore because I gained a lot of weight. Then I spent a lot of money on my CD collection. I now have 43 CDs."

"Oh my God!" said Roberta "That's a lot of CDs."

"Yes, it is," said Paisley. "I like different types of music. CDs take up a lot less storage space than vinyl records."

"Why did you buy a computer?" asked Alex. "To write a personal ad?"

"No, I got it to write a novel," said Paisley matter-of-factly. "It was actually a gift from my brother Plaid Jubilee. He is a lawyer in Washington, D.C."

"How is your novel doing?" asked Steven.

"Not very well so far," said Paisley. "But I'm working on it."

"You could include a condom with each copy," said Alex.

"That's enough of that," said Steven. "So how would you meet someone that you could take a trip to Florida with?"

"I met my last girlfriend at Overbrook," said Alex.

"That's a great idea, Alex," said Paisley. "Meet your significant other by getting yourself committed to a mental hospital."

"Well,' she turned out to be more of an insignificant other," said Alex, (emphasizing the "in" in "insignificant.") "If you know what I mean."

"I don't consider meeting someone in a mental hospital as the best way to meet someone," said Steven.

"You're probably right," agreed Paisley. "Maybe you could meet someone in jail."

"Or in Delaney Hall?" said Liza. Delaney Hall was an alternative to a women's prison in Newark. It was intended to be a place for ladies who did not commit violent crimes.

"Sometimes you just have to leave it in the hand of the lord," said Deanna. "He will provide for you."

"How do you meet someone who can have a relationship with?" asked Steven.

"I don't think I have a real true friend," said Priscilla "I used to have a lot of friends. I know a lot of people and I'm friendly with them, but they aren't really friends."

"How could you meet new friends?" asked Steven.

Across the hall in Room 4 was the Expression through Dancing Group. A boom box was playing Madonna singing "Material Girl."

"You can meet people many different ways," said Paisley. "You can meet people through a dating service."

"I've given up on dating," said Alex. "I've got too many problems to date. I don't have a job. I'm not in shape."

"Once you get hurt it won't happen again," said Priscilla. "I've learned through the pain of bad experiences."

"You can tell if someone is right for you by the chemistry between you," said Mary. "Once bitten twice shy."

"Do looks matter much to any of you?" asked Steven.

"It used to matter but now I know looks aren't everything," said Liza. "You have to take care of your life. There are a lot of potholes in a relationship. I play it by ear."

"Looks don't matter much," said Alex. "Someone can look fine but still be very sick. You can have HIV, syphilis and herpes and still look okay."

"People lie about these things. My ex-wife didn't tell me that she had herpes until after we were married," said Paisley. "So, we never tried to have intercourse."

"You have to have trust in the other person first," said Roberta. "Otherwise, there's nothing."

"There's a certain kind of social etiquette involved isn't there?" asked Steven.

"Yes, you don't walk up to a stranger and just say 'Let's go out,'" said Alex. "Well maybe you would if she had nice boobs."

"Oh yeah," responded Liza. "That's the most important thing!"

"That's enough of that," warned Steven. "Or I'll send you both to the director's office."

"You need to get to know someone first and then ask her to go out with you," said Mark. "She could be a psycho."

"You have to be sure a man is gay before you ask him to go out," said Paisley. "You can consider that as part of social etiquette."

"You can consider that as part of not being beaten up," said Alex. "A lot of men would be upset if a queer asked them out."

"I hadn't thought of that before," said Steven. "I guess gay men have to be more careful than straight men."

"Yes, they do," said Paisley "You don't want somcone to get angry at you."

"So how would you go about meeting someone?" asked Steven.

"You could go to a dance," said Priscilla. "That's how I met my first husband."

"You're right, Priscilla," said Paisley. "My parents met at a dance in Hartford, Connecticut many years ago."

"You could meet at church," said Roberta. "You usually meet good and kind people at any church."

"I go to lunch at churches on Saturdays," said Mark. "I guess you could meet new people that way."

"You could meet other people at work," said Steven. "I have made friends with some of my co-workers here."

"You can meet people just about anywhere," said Paisley. "I know a couple who met on the New York subway, and they've been together for more than ten years.

You can meet at bus stops, laundromats, even online at the supermarket."

"What do you say to these people?" asked Steven.

"Didn't I serve time with you in prison?" said Alex.

"Really now what do you say to strangers?" asked Steven.

"Well, you could start out by saying 'good morning' to them," said Paisley. "After you have seen this person on the bus several times you might start a conversation with them."

"You could meet someone at the gym," said Alex.

"After you meet someone what do you do with them?" asked Steven.

"You could to a game with them," said Mark. "You could go out to dinner with them."

"You could go to Six Flags, or Seaside Heights," said Priscilla. "There are a lot of things you can do on a date with someone."

From across the hall another song could be heard with the thumping bass. It was the song called "I'll Be Good to You" by the Brothers Johnson.

"I love that song they're playing now," said Liza.

She started humming the tune to herself. Then Alex and Mark started humming the same song too.

"The best thing is to meet someone through a friend like at a party or on a blind date," said Paisley. "Or a wedding."

"I hate blind dates," said Alex. "Especially if they bring their dog with them."

"I don't like the bar scene," said Priscilla. "They're smoke filled and everyone there just wants a one-night stand. With all the diseases out there, I have no interest in them."

"Are you involved with anyone now?" asked Alex.

"No, but if you want Alex, we can go to Connecticut and get married," said Paisley.

"Or maybe Vermont," said Alex.

"Are you gay?" asked Priscilla.

"No, I'm not," said Alex. "But I met some queers when I was in jail in Texas."

"They were just kidding," said Liza. "There were some lesbians at Delaney Hall when I was there."

"How come you don't like women?" asked Priscilla.

"How come you don't?" asked Paisley.

"I'm not attracted to them," said Priscilla.

"Neither am I," said Paisley.

"I think that people are born gay or straight," said Liza "My mother disagrees with me on that, like almost everything else."

"I don't care about that," said Alex. "I don't see why people make such a big deal about homosexuality anyway."

"Do you think it's harder to have a gay relationship?" asked Steven.

"Only the prejudice of others makes it harder," said Paisley. "In some ways it's easier. You don't have to worry about anybody getting pregnant or ever needing an abortion. If you're the same size, you can share clothes. You know what feels good to you, so you do the same thing to him."

"I never thought of that before," said Priscilla.

"Another way to meet people is to join social clubs," said Paisley. "Like a garden club, a knitting club, a bowling league. Something like that."

"Going out can be expensive," said Mark. "Dinner, and movies, these things cost money."

"I know," said Alex. "I remember when a phone call was just ten cents."

"I remember when they had telephone booths," said Paisley. "And they had cigarette vending machines in restaurants. My mother used to have me get cigarettes. She always smoked Parliaments. I once pulled the lever, and two packs came out at once."

"I remember when a postage stamp only cost twelve cents," said Mary.

"I remember when a blow job from a prostitute only cost ten dollars," said Alex, with an emphasis on "dollars."

"You have a disgusting mind," said Paisley. "I like that in a man."

"Thank you, Paisley," said Alex laughing. "If I was gay, would you go out with me?"

Paisley did not answer his question. The conversation stopped for a few minutes.

"What else do you like in someone else?" asked Steven, changing the subject intentionally.

"Money, lots of money," said Paisley. "I'm only joking. I like a man with a good sense of humor. Especially if he doesn't use illegal drugs."

"I do too," said Priscilla. "You've got a good point there, Paisley. My first husband Irving had a great sense of humor."

"So, what do you all plan on doing this weekend?" asked Steven.

"Get really, really drunk," said Alex who was M.I.C.A. "Or go to an AA meeting."

"You don't mean that do you?" asked Steven, obviously concerned.

"No, I don't. That was a bad joke," said Alex.

"I hope you're joking, Alex," said Roberta. "I don't want anything bad to happen to you that'll make you end up in jail again."

"You were in jail?" asked Priscilla.

"Yes, for one very long year in Texas," answered Alex. "I don't like to talk about it that much."

"I'm going to have some friends come over to play Yahtzee and Scrabble," said Paisley. "Then we'll order a pizza for dinner and some diet soda because I'm diabetic."

"I'm going to visit my sister," said Priscilla.

"Does anyone else have weekend plans?" asked Steven.

"I'm going out with my friends," said Roberta. "We're going to see that new Disney movie."

"I'm going to watch the game on TV," said Mark. "I hope my team wins."

"Who is your team?" asked Steven.

"I like the Yankees," said Mark.

"The Yankees suck," said Alex. "You're a fool."

"Fuck you," said Mark.

"I was kidding, kiddo," said Alex.

"Whatever!" yelled Mark "You're a bastard!"

"Okay everyone. The bell just rang so you can all go to your home groups now," said Steven. "Take care. Stay calm."

"You too, Steven," said Roberta. Roberta left the room humming her favorite hymn which was *A Mighty Fortress is Our God.*

Chapter 16

Over the years that he had been attending Campbell Care, Paisley had gone to at least a dozen different groups. Some reflected the interests of the counselor who ran it. Some were suggested by the patients themselves. The only thing for sure was that any group with less than six regular people attending would get cancelled. Everyone was reminded that people sleeping in boring groups was unacceptable because the officials from Medicaid might show up. They only allowed groups for people who were actively participating in them.

One of the groups that Paisley liked, besides the Human Sexuality group, was the Storytelling Group. It was often unpredictable how it would be because the attendees had to contribute original ideas to it. This group was run by a nice 40-year-old white woman named Sharon.

Sharon was a very talented lady. She was not only a wonderful counselor, with an M.A. in psychology but was also a musician who could play both the piano and the guitar beautifully. She was the only counselor at Campbell Care who could play musical instruments and was also a certified music therapist. Therefore, she also ran a very popular group called Music Therapy which Paisley did not attend himself.

This group had a good selection of people in it. There was Lois, Alex, Liza, Mary, Carlos, Annie, Joy, and Kenneth. Carlos was a 26-year-old Peruvian man with lustrous black hair. He always wore white shirts and black pants that were somewhat baggy but still showed off his nice shape. Paisley would never tell him that he was attractive because his personality was like his plain clothes, being somewhat conservative. Yet he liked Paisley to feel his shaven face sometimes.

As was often the case, Paisley was one of the first people to enter Room 4 where the Storytelling group was always held. Other people came into the room and sat down in an assortment of chairs all donations to Campbell Care from various sources. One of the differences between the Storytelling Group and other groups was that everyone was required to participate in this group.

Nobody could lazily sleep through this group as they did in the Medication Education group. Everybody was called upon to add their input to the short story which was composed during this therapy group. Each person was asked as they went around the room to contribute something to the story which was the result of every storytelling group. It was one group where all the participants could use their imagination as well, instead of depending on facts about different subjects such as paranoid schizophrenia, which was the diagnosis of most patients at Campbell Care.

Sharon entered the room and sat in the chair nearest to the white door which led into the room. She always brought a plastic tote bag containing music CDs that she would sometimes play during the group for patients' inspiration.

"Hi, everybody! How are you all doing?" asked Sharon cheerfully.

"Okay, thank God," said Joy. "The father, the son and the holy spirit. I think Jesus will be coming back soon."

"I'm alright," said Lois. "But Sharon do you think parents can conceal a divorce from their children? Is that really possible?"

"I don't know why they would want to do that in the first place Lois," said Sharon. "I guess it's possible to do that."

"They might want to keep small children from finding out about it," said Carlos.

"That's true," said Lois. "I forgot about that."

"Where should we begin today's story?" asked Sharon.

"Jesus will come back soon and clean house," said Joy.

Joy usually carried a large black bag with her. It always contained something that she was knitting. She claimed that she found knitting to be very relaxing.

"Thank you, Joy," said Sharon.

"I'll start," said Mary.

Sharon wrote down everything that everyone said and often repeated it afterward before the group ended. The finished product was never the same from week to week. However, sometimes the story was simply weak.

"There's a beautiful meadow where deer and rabbits are running around," said Mary. "There are butterflies flying in the air."

"There are all types of beautiful flowers," said Lois. "We are in the year 1960. Two people named John and Maryann are walking through a mountain trail in Vermont."

"Why Vermont?" asked Carlos. "Why not Maine?"

"I love Vermont for a great vacation," sang Lois.

Lois was imitating an old commercial which suggested Vermont as an ideal place for a visit.

"I think Vermont is okay, Lois," said Alex. "That's where Paisley and I are going to get married soon."

"Since when did you decide that?" asked Sharon, missing Alex's frequently sarcastic tone.

"I know nothing about this," said Paisley "I'm totally blown away. I don't remember you ever even asking me to go to Vermont with you."

"Exactly," said Alex. "That's the point."

"Yeah, and I'm not going to be the maid of honor!" said Liza.

"I don't know if two men could ever get married," said Joy to no one's surprise, including Paisley himself. "I thought the bible says two men and two women can't get married."

"Whatever," said Sharon. "Maybe that will change some day. Particularly since this is the 21st Century."

Sharon may have been clearly in disagreement with Joy. Being neutral like Switzerland, she did not want to start a dispute over sexual politics. Her job was to keep everyone focused on the work at hand, and not to discuss the Bible.

"I'm not worried about that at all."

"You're not, Sharon?" asked Carlos. "You should be."

"No, I'm not," said Sharon. "Alex must be joking."

"Marry whomever you want is what I believe," said Liza. "Screw the Republicans!"

"Do you still think parents could conceal a divorce?" asked Lois one last time. "Is that possible, Sharon?"

"No, it is not," said Liza. "My parents got divorced and I knew all about it. My mother got married a second time and then divorced him. My stepfather sends me money for my birthday sometimes."

"That's so nice, Liza," said Sharon.

"Why are you so concerned about divorce, Lois?" asked Kenneth. "Are you going to get a divorce, Lois?"

"I've never been married," said Lois. "Have you, Kenneth?"

"No, I haven't Lois," said Kenneth. "I would never marry my lover."

"You had a lover?" asked Carlos, smiling at Kenneth. "I didn't know you were gay."

"I am gay Carlos," admitted Kenneth. "Do you have a problem with that?"

"No, I don't," said Carlos. "Just as long as you don't make a pass at me."

"I don't want ever to get married," said Lois. "I'm too old now any way."

"Who would want to marry you?" asked Mary.

"That's pretty weird," said Carlos.

"Speaking of pretty weird," said Sharon. "Let's get back to our story. Alex you're next to add something to our magnum opus."

"They go beside a babbling book. They parked their two-toned convertible by the street," said Alex.

"My parents had a convertible," said Lois. "It was blue and white."

"What happened to your parents?" asked Carlos.

"They're both deceased. My father died in 2003 and my mother died in 2006 right after she had a big party for my fiftieth birthday on September 5, 2006," said Lois.

"Okay, Carlos it's your turn now," said Sharon.

"They left the parade that was coming down the street to get some peace and quiet in nature," said Carlos, as Sharon continued writing.

"What parade was it?" asked Lois. "The Easter Parade?"

"The Gay Pride Parade," said Liza.

"They didn't have gays in 1960," said Lois. "I mean they didn't have Gay Pride Parades in 1960, did they? I think one of the girls in high school back then was like that."

"Maybe they did in Denmark," said Alex. "That's always been a liberal country."

"Christine Jorgensen came from Denmark," said Lois.

"She went abroad and came back a broad," said Alex.

"Oh lord can we tear ourselves away from this stuff?" asked Sharon. "Let's return to our unfinished story about John and Maryann, please?"

"John fell asleep under a tree and Maryann sat quietly reading a book," said Joy. "It was a book about knitting."

"Very good, Joy," said Sharon, writing in her notebook.

"What kind of tree did he fall asleep under?" asked Lois. "Was it a weeping willow?"

"No Lois," said Liza. "It was poison sumac."

"It doesn't matter," said Sharon. "Liza, please don't upset Lois."

"If it was a poison sumac tree, John might get a rash," said Lois. "A magnolia tree would be pleasing."

"John dreamed about the army he fought in," said Alex continuing the story. "He thought of his friend that died in the war. When he awakened from the dream, he realized how lucky he was to be alive."

"What war was he in?" asked Lois. "The war of the roses?"

"The War of the Roses," said Alex.

"My mother's favorite flower was roses," said Lois. "She preferred pink roses. I loved to get flowers when I was a young girl."

"My mother's favorite song was, 'Red Roses for a Blue Lady' And no, I don't know who wrote it, Lois," added Paisley anticipating her usual questions. "Look it up on the Internet next time you go to the library with your social worker."

"You're next Kenneth," said Sharon. "Go ahead."

"Maryann wasn't John's first finance," continued Kenneth. "Maryann didn't know it but John had an affair with Collette when he was at war. He never told Mary about Colette, but Collette had his baby."

"So, John was an adulterer then?" asked Annie.

"Yes, I guess he was an adulterer," said Paisley.

"No, he wasn't an adulterer," said Alex.

"Well, he certainly wasn't an adulteress," said Lois. "Because an adulteress is a woman."

"He wasn't married to his finance Maryann yet," said Alex. "So, he wasn't really an adulterer legally."

Paisley took a sip from his can of diet cherry Coke. He looked from Kenneth to Liza. All three of them started laughing. Liza made a gesture with her left hand like someone holding a telephone. Paisley nodded "Yes" at her meaning that he would call her later that day.

"It's your turn Mary," said Sharon.

Throughout everyone's recitation of the story, Sharon continued writing what everyone contributed to the silly short story. She sometimes rolled her hazel eyes and smiled gently.

"Then he was just a good-for-nothing two timing womanizer," said Mary. "That's why Maryann divorced her first husband. He had an affair with her best friend, Sally Newman."

"That must have been a terrible situation for Maryann," said Sharon. "I know I would have felt a sense of betrayal, if I ever found out someone did that to me. Has anyone else had something like this ever happen to them?"

"I had a girlfriend in Peru who did a good one on me," said Carlos.

"What do you mean by that?" asked Sharon.

"She put a spell on me," said Carlos. "She used witchcraft on me. That's why I have emotional problems."

"God wouldn't let that happen to you," said Joy. "I don't believe in that sort of thing."

"That's just a lot of superstitious bullshit," said Liza. "Even if the devil was a woman, no bitch can put a spell on you. She could try to get you high as a kite though."

"Liza, that is not a nice word," said Sharon. "Okay Joy it's your turn."

"The baby's name was Lois," said Joy. "The baby talked a lot. That's all I have to say this time."

Joy continued knitting a sapphire-colored blanket. Several people at Campbell Care offered to pay Joy a commission to knit something for them. So far, she had refused all of their offers.

"John was attracted to Maryann because she reminded him of Collette," said Paisley. "John finally tells Maryann about Collette and the baby."

"Was there anything in your life that led you to say that Paisley?" asked Sharon.

"Yes, there was," answered Paisley. "I had a real-life situation where I met someone who looked exactly like someone else."

"They say that everyone has a twin out there somewhere," said Alex. "You must have met someone's twin."

"I was living in Albany, New York at the time," said Paisley. "I went to a bar and met a guy who looked just like my first boyfriend, Dominick. The next morning, he saw a photo of Dominick and said something that I'll never forget. He said, 'Where did you get that picture of me'?"

"I guess the guy was your type, dude," said Kenneth.

"Have anyone here ever seen the movie directed by Alfred Hitchcock called 'Vertigo'?" asked Alex. "It's really cool."

"No, I haven't," said Sharon.

"Well, the main character was played by James Stewart," said Alex.

"I always liked James Cagney," interrupted Lois. "He won an Oscar for my favorite movie 'Yankee Doodle Dandy.'"

"You are being very rude, Lois," said Sharon. "Alex was talking Lois."

"I'm sorry," said Lois.

"James Stewart met a woman who looked like another woman exactly," said Alex. "He fell in love with the second woman only because she looked like his first old lady who had passed away."

"That's very interesting, Alex," said Paisley. "Alfred Hitchcock is one of my favorite directors. I'm surprised he never won an Oscar."

"I know about a lot of people who should have gotten Oscars but never did," said Alex. "Barbara Stanwyck, Sammy Davis Jr., Mamie Van Doren, and Cary Grant."

"That is all very interesting," said Sharon. "Now Liza can you continue our story?"

"Maryann isn't really upset after all. She decides to adopt the baby because Colette was no longer around. Colette tripping off magic mushrooms threw herself off the Eiffel tower. John, Maryann, and Lois lived happily ever after. The End."

"Thank you, Liza," said Sharon. "That was a good though dramatic and traumatic end to our tale. Why did you have Colette throw herself off the Eiffel Tower? Are you feeling suicidal?"

"No, I'm not feeling suicidal now," said Liza. "I just felt like it. I have never been to Paris however."

"I hope not," said Sharon. "I would have to send you to crisis otherwise."

Crisis was the part of the hospital where people were sent if they said that they were feeling suicidal. Another reason to be sent there was if someone felt homicidal. While they were there, the staff would decide whether the person's situation was serious enough to require admission to the psychiatric ward.

They usually made sick people remove their belts and shoelaces to prevent someone from hanging himself or herself. They would ask several questions to see if the person was disoriented or not. Questions like what year it was, who was the president, and such.

If the patient stayed there long enough, he or she might be sent to a permanent mental hospital like Overbook or Greystone. Paisley's friend Jim had been sent to Greystone for two years.

"Has anyone here even felt suicidal like Collette in the story?" asked Sharon.

"Yes, I have," said Paisley. "After my mother died, I attempted suicide by taking an overdose of pills."

"God says committing suicide is a sin," said Joy. "You'll go to hell Paisley."

"Or at least purgatory," said Annie. "I felt that way after my mother died. It was right before they hit the World Trade Center."

"You don't feel that way now do you, Annie?" asked Sharon quite seriously.

"Heavens no, Sharon," said Annie. "I am on antidepressants now that control 'suicidal ideations' as Dr. Patel calls them. My life isn't perfect, but I don't want to end it."

"I want to live so that I can continue writing," said Paisley. "Dead men cannot write novels."

"Dead men cannot write novels," repeated Alex. "That sounds like the title for a movie directed by John Carpenter."

"Really now," said Liza. "That might make a good Stephen King story."

"If you really write a novel, Paisley, I'd like to read it," said Kenneth.

"I'd like to read it too," said Sharon.

"Thank you," said Paisley. "I've already started writing a novel. It's called 'Fake Face.'"

"That's a cool name," said Sharon. "I never heard of any book called that before."

"I like that name too," said Alex. "It's really catchy, because it's so easy to remember."

"It sure is," said Sharon. "Do you want me to read back what we've written today?"

"Let's do that next week," said Mary looking at her watch. "The coffee break is about to start."

Paisley looked up at the round white clock with black numbers like all the other clocks at Campbell Care. It read 10:49. The bell rang just as Paisley, glanced at the clock. The ending of this period was the beginning of the first fifteen-minute break of this day.

Everyone left Room 4 and headed right down the hall to the APR where coffee was being given out. Lois firmly grasped her large plastic coffee mug which was brown and said 'Dunkin Donuts' on it.

"I can't wait to read your book," said Sharon.

"Thank you," said Paisley. "And tell all your friends to buy it too."

"Absolutely," said Sharon sincerely.

Paisley wove his way through the people lining up to get coffee. He then exited the double doors that led to the Campbell Care parking lot. Some people were already outside smoking cigarettes. Paisley passed Jim standing alone outside of the small warehouse attached by a large breezeway to the main building. Jim almost always stood there unless he was talking to Kenneth who only attended Campbell Care on Mondays, Wednesdays, and Thursdays.

"Hi, Jim," said Paisley.

"Hi, Paisley," said Jim. "I have some bad news to tell you."

"What is it?"

"My boarding home is going to be sold in two months. So, I'll have to move," said Jim calmly.

At first Paisley felt fine and then a dread passed over him.

"Where will you move to? Another boarding home?"

"No, I decided that this is as good a time as any to do something I've always thought of doing."

"What is that?" asked Paisley fearing Jim's answer.

"I'm going to move down south to live with my mother. All my brothers and sisters live down there too and I miss them."

"Will you stay in touch with me?"

"Of course, I will Paisley," said Jim looking directly into Paisley eyes.

"Okay."

Paisley felt like crying but held his sorrow at check. He slowly walked to Happy Pharmacy and bought two cans of diet cherry Coke, putting them into his tote bag. Coming back, he looked at the warehouse, but Jim was no longer there. Paisley would have to get used to seeing no one there soon if Jim really did move down south.

However, as Paisley looked skyward the sun came out of the clouds and shone into his eyes. Like a light in the darkness of his soul an idea hit him with the sunbeam. It was an idea that Paisley never thought of before. Paisley realized that he may have found the solution to his fear of forever losing Jim. Paisley would simply move down south with Jim!

"Of course, why not?" asked Paisley of himself out loud. "But would Jim allow me to do that?"

Chapter 17

Paisley really wanted to see Kenneth and Jim outside of Campbell Care. He had already discussed visiting Liza at her mother's house in Cedar Grove. He wanted to see her alone for the time being. At their program, Jim, Kenneth, and Paisley all seemed to be very compatible with each other. It also appeared that they would be able to spend time together on their own, beyond the structured setting of Campbell Care. Being with two people whom he already knew Paisley assumed that Kenneth's anxiety level would be well under control.

The date was set for that Saturday at noon. They all agreed to meet at the McDonald's restaurant inside Newark Penn Station. It was the hub where all the choices for transportation met. There were the PATH trains, the Newark light rail, the New Jersey Transit trains to Manhattan, the Greyhound bus lines, and the Amtrak trains that Paisley took to see his brother and sister-in-law for Christmas in Connecticut.

After taking a cool shower, Paisley put on some plain white briefs, a green T-shirt, and a pair of blue and black plaid shorts. He sat on the edge of his twin bed and pulled on a pair of green socks and then slipped his diabetic feet into a pair of brown Rockport shoes. His foot doctor had informed him those diabetics should never wear tight shoes. The circulation was already a little sluggish in his feet and uncomfortable shoes could cause blisters that could become infected easily. Because Paisley remembered that his mother had not taken very good care of her own diabetic feet, he did not want to follow in her footsteps.

Mental illness could be a dense fog for some people. Voices can be heard in the distance, but you cannot see who is speaking. Shadows and shapes move through the mist. You can't tell if they are there or not. The right medication can cut through the fog and slowly you are aware of yourself, as if you were a blind man seeing his own face for the first time.

Paisley looked at himself in his bathroom mirror. He combed his graying auburn hair with a tortoise shell type comb that his sister-in-law had placed in his Christmas stocking the year before. He parted his hair on the right side because the wave in his hair fell naturally in that direction. His friends had often commented on his wavy and thick hair ever since he was a teenager.

Paisley made sure that he had his house keys with him, before he left his apartment. He removed the Prado Museum tote bag from the doorknob on his living room closet. He locked the front door before getting onto the elevator. He pressed the metal button on the wall in the hallway between the two elevator doors. A little bell inside the walls rang right as the right-hand elevator doors opened. He did not check his mail in the little mailroom in the lobby, because he thought it would have nothing but bills in it. He had left the Easter Seals place to get his one bedroom apartment. He left his twelve-story apartment building and walked three blocks to the Branch Brook Park light rail station. He took the train to the last stop which was Penn Station.

Both Jim and Kenneth were waiting near McDonald's just as they had planned beforehand.

"Hi, Jim. Hi, Kenneth."

"Hi, Paisley," said both Jim and Kenneth at the same time.

"Was that in stereophonic sound?" asked Paisley. "You both said 'Hi Paisley' in unison."

"Oh yeah, you're right," said Jim.

"Maybe it was an echo," answered Kenneth laughingly.

Jim and Kenneth were dressed in their usual attire. Kenneth was wearing a gray long sleeved shirt, black pants, and black shoes. He rarely wore bright colors like red or orange. Jim was wearing a maroon polo shirt, blue jeans, and blue sneakers. Because Jim was six feet tall and a little chunky around the middle, he had to buy his clothes at one of those specialty shops for tall men.

"We need to take the PATH train now," said Paisley. "First I need to get some money out of the Bank of America ATM machine."

"I have thirty dollars," said Jim. "Is that going to be enough?"

"Yeah, don't worry about it, dude," said Kenneth. "I have extra money because I work one day a week for Project Live."

"What do you do?" asked Jim.

"Mostly maintenance work on Project Live houses," answered Kenneth.

"I just hope that the PATH trains are running okay," said Paisley.

"What do you mean?" asked Kenneth anxiously. "Now I wonder if we should go there today."

"Don't worry about it," said Jim. "I think it sometimes runs slow on the weekend."

They walked from McDonald's to the long corridor which led to the huge main lobby on the right and the PATH train and public restrooms on the left. There were also several shops there: Hudson News, Liquor Store, Zarro's bakery, and Yummy Pizza.

"One time when I took the PATH train it was so late that I missed the train I wanted to take to Upstate New York to visit my friend Michael McPartlin. So, I had to come back. Then the train stopped running at Harrison, NJ."

They entered the glass door leading to the escalator which went to the PATH train platform. That was also where the vending machines were to buy PATH train tickets. It was easy to identify them because they had the purple, blue, and orange PATH logo on the front of them.

"Oh shit, Paisley," said Kenneth. "I heard enough, okay?"

"That almost never happens," said Jim calmly.

The three of them got into line at one of the three vending machines. They each inserted $2.75 to buy a one-way ticket to Manhattan. Then they placed their tickets into the slot on the front of the turnstiles that gave you access to the PATH train platform. A little screen said, "Card captured. Enter now." After Jim, Kenneth, and Paisley entered the three turnstiles, they found one of the chrome metal benches on which to sit and wait for the next PATH train.

"How long do you think we'll have to wait, Paisley?" asked Kenneth.

"I would guess about fifteen to twenty minutes. Then we have to switch trains at the Journal Square stop. We will cross the platform and catch the train going to 33rd Street in Manhattan."

"Are we going to 33rd Street?" asked Jim.

"No, we'll get out at 9th Street," answered Paisley.

There was a dozen or so people waiting on the platform. Some of them were talking on their cell phones. Most of them were couples or groups of three or four people. The ones with children were probably families going to The Big Apple for a daytrip. No matter what day or time Paisley had taken the PATH trains over the last decade the platform was never completely full. Perhaps some people worked later shifts on the weekdays.

There were not just people on the platform. Occasionally a pigeon or sparrow would fly into the station. Both ends of the platform opened onto the outside. Birds would dart into the station and peck at little crumbs of food on the platform. You could easily tell that birds had been there because sometimes there was a donut that someone had dropped with lots of marks in it. They were probably made from hungry birds pecking at them.

"Thank god those are only pigeons," said Paisley.

"What do you mean?" asked Jim.

"Just imagine if those were ostriches instead," said Paisley. "Could you see big ostriches running up and down the platform eating the donuts that someone dropped?"

"You're really weird, dude," said Kenneth. "What the fuck made you think of ostriches? Those things live in Australia. That's thousands of miles from New Jersey."

"Yeah, but those big birds lay eggs that could feed all three of us for a week," said Jim.

"I never thought of that before," said Kenneth. "Hey, Paisley, do you think that dude is one of us?"

"Who do you mean? Oh, the black guy with the pink hoodie on?" asked Paisley. "Maybe his girlfriend gave it to him."

"I hope nobody thinks I'm gay," said Jim. "Just because you said that."

"As long as we don't hold hands, nobody will think that," said Kenneth, laughing.

"You two aren't you know—" said Jim.

"No, we aren't lovers," said Paisley interrupting what Jim was asking. "Kenneth and I are just friends. He and I discussed that already. I'm not his type."

"Oh alright," said Jim. "I'm sorry I said that."

"I don't mind you asking that," said Paisley. "I have had that discussion with all of my gay male friends about whether we're just friends or not. I mean you have female friends who aren't your girlfriends, right?"

"I see what you mean," said Jim.

A PATH train came to the station finally. The lights and the rushing noise grew louder and then ended as the train stopped at the platform. Jim, Kenneth, and Paisley got up from the bench where they had been sitting and entered one of the cars. They sat to the right of the open doors in a seat that could hold only the three of them. Kenneth preferred not to sit next to strangers whenever it was possible.

A little while later a voice over the intercoms said, "Please watch the closing doors." There were a few beeps and then the doors closed.

At both ends of the cars were little digital screens attached to the ceiling. They were long and rectangular with red letters on a black background. The message read "Next Stop Journal Square."

"Have you ever taken this train all the way to Manhattan?" asked Jim.

"No, never," replied Paisley. "We always have to switch trains at Journal Square. Then the train goes to Hoboken, Grove Street, Christopher Street, 9th Street, 14th, 23rd and 33rd Streets. We usually get out at 9th Street."

"The 9th Street is on Sixth Avenue," said Kenneth. "We always go to the Gay Center and meet friends there."

"The Center is on West 13th Street," added Paisley.

"Oh yeah, I met you there once, didn't I?" asked Jim. "It's right across from a church where I've gone to get a free lunch."

"Where do you want to eat lunch?" asked Paisley. "It doesn't matter to me."

"Any place that has meat," said Kenneth. "No sushi or vegetarian places for me."

"We could go to the French Bistro," suggested Paisley. "I've been there a million times. I even went there once with my mother about twenty years ago."

The train stopped at Harrison. About ten minutes later it stopped at Journal Square. Everybody got off of the PATH train to wait for the 33rd Street train to Manhattan.

"Oh wow, look at that!" said Paisley.

"Look at what?" asked Kenneth.

"There's a woman at the end of this car reading a book called 'Strange Justice,' written by Jill Abramson," said Paisley.

"Who is Jill Abramson?" asked Kenneth. "Do you know her or what, dude?"

"Yes, I know her," answered Paisley. "She is one of my brother and sister-in-law's best friends. That book is kind of old though. It was published during the end of the 20th Century."

"That's cool," said Jim. "Did they make a movie out of it?"

"I don't know," said Paisley. "I'll have to ask them next time I go there for Christmas."

The train reached Journal Square and the three friends exited the train to wait on the platform. Because both ends of the station were open to the outdoors, there was a cool breeze blowing through the platform. It was a Saturday near the end of October. In winter it was usually a very brisk wind which deterred Paisley from going to Manhattan then. The PATH train to 33rd Street, arrived about fifteen minutes later.

Kenneth grabbed a seat that fit only the three of them again. The second half of the trip took about an hour. The train stopped at Hoboken and Grove Street before heading thru the tunnel which connected New Jersey to New York. Paisley actually knew a friend who commuted from New Jersey to New York every weekday, as did multitudes of other professional men and women.

After leaving the long tunnel under the Hudson River, the PATH stopped at Christopher Street. Christopher Street had been a very popular gay destination in the 1970s and

1980s, before AIDS and gentrification made Greenwich Village too expensive for gay men and artists to live there. A sign of times was when The Oscar Wilde Memorial Bookstore on the corner of Gay and Christopher Streets went out of business. It had become a dress shop for well-to-do women. Some of the former gay bars had closed and now sold baby clothes to upper class young couples.

Because it was a week before Halloween, store windows were decked out with pictures of skeletons, vampires, and witches.

"Why don't we go to the restaurant first, and then see if there are any movies showing at Quad Cinema afterward," said Paisley.

They ascended three sets of stairs until they reached the street level. The train tunnels produced a kind of vacuum effect, causing a very strong breeze to blow on them while they walked up the stairways. Across the street from the 9th Street exit was a Hard Rock Café on the corner of 6th Avenue. On the opposite side of 6th Avenue was a fenced in little community garden which was next to an old library. It had a tower in it with a large clock.

The restaurant was on the corner of 6th Avenue and West 11th Street. There was a copy of the menu posted on the front window next to the main entrance.

"This doesn't look too expensive," said Kenneth. "Okay we can go here for lunch."

They went into The French Bistro thru the wooden double doors. The place was full of nice round tables. On the far right was a bar with stools lined up in front of it. A set of stairs lead to a smaller room on the left side of the main dining room. There were pictures on the wall of sites in Paris like the Eiffel Tower. They were copies of posters designed by the famous artist Henri de Toulouse Lautrec as well.

A pretty waitress in a black dress approached them.

"Can I help you gentlemen?"

"Yes, we would like a table for three, please," said Paisley politely.

She led them to a large table with four matching wooden chairs around it.

"Here you are."

"Merci, mademoiselle," said Paisley.

Paisley sat on one chair and placed his Prado Museum tote bag on the white chair next to him. Kenneth sat between Paisley and Jim.

Because the restaurant was on a busy street like 7th Avenue, they could see all sorts of people walking up and down the avenue. There were large windows in the corner of the restaurant through which to see them. A young white woman with a black leather jacket, a white shirt, and pink hair passed the window.

"Oh God!" said Paisley. "Did you see her?"

"You mean that girl with the pink hair?" asked Kenneth.

"Yes, I do," said Paisley. "I haven't seen anyone like that since 1982."

"What comes around, goes around," said Jim.

"Are you ready to order gentleman?" asked a Spanish waiter. "Or should I come back in a few minutes?"

"Could you come back?" said Paisley. "Thank you."

They looked over the menus and stopped talking for a few moments. The entrees were priced around $15 or more, which was reasonable for a restaurant in Manhattan.

The same waiter returned shortly and said, "Are you ready now?"

"Yes, I'd like the chicken Cesar salad," said Paisley. "And I'd also like a glass of diet coke with a twist of lemon in it, please."

"That sounds good," said Jim. "I'll have the same thing."

"I'll have the Bistro burger well done," said Kenneth. "And I'd like a regular coke with that."

The waiter finished writing down their orders.

"Is this all together?"

"No, we'll have separate checks this time," said Kenneth.

Paisley noticed Kenneth watching the waiter walk away toward the kitchen.

"What are you looking at?" asked Paisley.

"What do you think, dude?" replied Kenneth, laughingly.

"This is a nice place, Paisley," said Jim. "I'm glad we came here."

"I was hoping that you two gentlemen would like it too," said Paisley. "I've been here a few times before."

"How long has this place been here?" asked Kenneth.

"I don't know, but I would guess about ten years or so."

"That's a pretty long time for New York," said Jim.

The waiter brought their drinks to the round table with the gingham tablecloth.

"Thank you," said Paisley.

"Yeah, places come and go in this city so fast," said Jim. "It must be hard to make a restaurant successful in such a competitive place like New York."

"If you can make it here you can make it anywhere," sang Paisley. "It's up to you, New York, New York."

"Frank Sinatra?" asked Jim. "Right?"

"Yes, he sang that old tune," said Paisley.

Paisley sipped his cool drink. It felt almost as refreshing as a dip into the ocean.

"If it's older than you, it must be old," said Kenneth.

"Yeah right," sneered Paisley playfully. "You're a year older than me, you bastard."

"I'm older than both of you," said Jim. "And I am about to become a grandfather."

"Oh wow," said Paisley. "Congratulations. Does becoming a grandfather really make you feel old?"

"Yes, it does," replied Jim. "But I can handle it."

The Spanish waiter brought Kenneth's Bistro burger to him and placed it on the table.

"Thank you," said Kenneth. "Now this is real food for real men."

"What? I thought you were a vegetarian," said Paisley.

"Me? A vegetarian?" asked Kenneth, holding his burger. "Never in a million years. I eat vegetarians."

The waiter then brought Paisley and Jim their chicken Cesar salads and placed them in front of them.

"This looks delicious," said Paisley.

"That's not all," said Kenneth, whose gaze followed the waiter across the room. "I think I know what I want for dessert too."

"What does that mean?" asked Jim. "Oh yeah the waiter. I prefer the hostess that showed us to our table."

"You dirty old man!" said Kenneth. "And you a grandfather?"

"How do you think he became a grandfather anyway?" said Paisley. "Or do you still think that the stork brings babies?"

They all stopped talking a few minutes while they enjoyed themselves by eating their food. Being good friends, they did not feel that something was wrong if the conversation ever lulled. In fact, Paisley preferred friends who were more taciturn than loquacious.

"Do you want to go to the Quad and see what is playing there after lunch, guys?" asked Paisley.

"Sure, that would be good," said Jim. "I like their movies except for the ones where I have to read subtitles because the movies in Tagalog or something."

"I know what you mean dude," said Kenneth. "And no more weird French movies where the Virgin Mary works at a gas station."

"Okay, no more wasting money on bad French films," said Paisley. "I'll make a mental note of that."

After they finished their lunch and paid for their individual tabs, they left the Bistro Café. All they had to do was to walk north two blocks, and east one long block. The blocks between avenues were longer than the ones between the numbered streets.

"Here we are," said Paisley. He opened one of the double doors leading into the movie theater and held it for Kenneth. They looked at the posters on the walls and decided on a movie.

"How about this one?" asked Paisley. "It looks like a comedy."

"Which one do you mean?" asked Jim.

"This one called 'Turtle Hill, Brooklyn.' And it's in English. And it's new and was made in 2011."

"Alright, that's the one," said Kenneth. "Let's get our tickets and go sit down. No more movies that are older than you.:"

There was a small ticket window with a salesman sitting behind it. On the wall behind him was a board that listed the four movies showing in the theater that day, and the times that they all began.

They walked through the main doors past a row of round seats. A young black man wearing a black T-shirt that said "Quad Staff" stood at the entrance to the four small movie theaters inside the building.

"Tickets please," he said.

They showed him their ticket stubs.

"It's the first door on the left, theater one."

"Thank you," said Paisley.

They went into the dark theater which only had four people sitting in it already.

"Where should we sit?" asked Paisley.

"Not in the first or the last rows," said Kenneth.

"How about here?" said Jim, who was standing near the middle section.

"Alright this will do," said Paisley.

Kenneth went in first and sat down, followed by Paisley with Jim sitting in the seat on the aisle. There was only one aisle between two sets of seats in the small theater. Two signs saying "Exit" in red letters were near the front of the theater. There were two dim lights on the walls. When the movie started a few minutes later, the lights went dark.

The movie was only one and a half hours long. Because it was very funny, and well done, the time seemed to pass very quickly and pleasantly. It was a movie about several friends who lived in Brooklyn.

After the movie ended, the lights went up and the credits rolled. Then there was special surprise. The director of the movie itself was there.

"Hello, everybody. Did you like the movie? I am the director, Brian."

Someone said to him "Yes it was a very good movie, even though it was probably shot on a limited budget."

"Thank you," replied Brian, a handsome young man in his early thirties. "I am making low budget films now but hope to get more funding in the future."

"Is this movie based on a true story?" asked Kenneth.

"Yes, it was," answered Brian. "Many of my cast are also friends of mine who are willing to work for a low salary to help me out."

"Are you interested in any new projects?" asked Paisley. "I just finished writing a novel that might make a good movie."

"Is your book published yet?" asked Brian.

"No not yet, but I could give you a copy of it."

"Meet me in the lobby and we can discuss it more."

Paisley, Kenneth, and Jim left the theater. A few minutes later they were in the lobby. There was a folding wooden table set up with DVDs of the movie on it for sale.

"Would you like to buy a DVD?" asked a young woman who was in the movie they just saw.

"Yes, I would," said Paisley. "Do you think the director could autograph it for me?"

Brian just entered the room. "I have never been asked for my autograph before."

He removed the plastic cover and signed the paper cover underneath. He handed it to Paisley.

"Thank you," said Paisley. "I bet someday people will be asking for your autograph all the time."

"I would like to read your manuscript. What is it about?"

"It's about my life in the mental health system. Could I send you a printout of it?"

"Yes, here is my business card."

"My name is Paisley Jubilee, by the way."

They shook hands. Brian laughed.

"Is that your real name?"

"Yes, it is," said Jim. "Everyone asks him that. I read the manuscript and I think Paisley wrote a wonderful novel."

"I look forward to reading it," said Brian. "Here is my snail mail address to send the manuscript to me."

"Thank you, Brian," said Paisley warmly.

"Could there be a role in it for me?" asked the young brunette lady behind the table with the DVDs on it.

"Oh yes there are many female characters in the novel. Maybe you could play a therapist."

"Take care," said Brian. "After I read the novel, I'll send you an email."

"Goodbye," said Paisley as he, Jim and Kenneth left Quad Cinema.

"It's getting late," said Jim outside on 13th Street. "I want to check out a bookstore that sells science fiction books and comic books too."

"I think we'll pass on that," said Kenneth.

"Okay, I'll call you soon," said Paisley. "Good night."

"We'll see you again at program, dude," said Kenneth.

Jim walked away toward Fifth Avenue. Kenneth and Paisley went to Sixth Avenue and down to 9th Street to catch the PATH train back to Newark.

"I can't believe that guy wants to read your book," said Kenneth. "It would be really cool if he liked it and made a movie about it."

"Yes, it would be incredible to see my name in big letters on the screen. 'Based on a novel by Paisley Jubilee.'"

That night Paisley slept better than ever. The next day he mailed a copy of his novel *Fake Face* to Brian the director. He had never considered the possibility of having one of his novels as the basis for a film.

Chapter 18

Going to New York City with two of his friends gave him another impression of them. Whenever they were at Campbell Care, everything that they said and did could be observed by trained psychotherapists and social workers. Outside of that place, they could talk about other patients candidly, without the risk of causing a fight with anyone.

Paisley had some therapy groups that could be very interesting one day and then very boring on another day. This was not only dependent on the personality of the counselor who ran the groups but also on the patients who attended it as well. There were some patients who slept through group periods because they were heavily medicated. They were others who were pathologically shy and rarely participated in groups even if the topic of discussion seemed to be suited to them. Still other patients were so preoccupied with the voices inside their heads that they almost never spoke directly to anyone.

The group call Social Skills was that kind of group. Social Skills always took place in Room 2. It was a long room painted white with brown plastic chairs lining the walls. Room 2 had one feature unique to only it and Room 1. There was an emergency exit at the end of the room which could be opened to let in fresh air if the room ever seemed hot or stuffy. This was particularly true in the spring and summer months.

Paisley entered the room first and sat down at a chair next to a brown table at the right end of the room. After the bell rang, other patients filled the room. They were Mark, Kenneth who was Paisley's Scrabble partner, Gino, Annie, Mary, Priscilla, Joy, Kevin, and Jason. Jim was the last patient to enter the room. He sat down next to Paisley as he always did. His right arm brushed against Paisley's left one and Paisley felt a jolt of electricity race up and down his spine. Paisley wondered if Jim ever knew how good he made him feel with the slightest touch or glance.

Jose the counselor finally came into Room 2 and sat down in the only yellow chair in the room. It was the one nearest the gray door which was the entrance to the room. He was always very pleasant and usually wore plaid shirts and blue jeans that were neither tight nor too loose.

The clothing of most of the staff members was usually casual. None of the counselors ever wore designer fashions or much makeup. Paisley remembered that he had been told once that the staff probably did not make enough money to afford such things. The only people who ever wore better clothes were the assistant director, and her boss who was the director of Campbell Care.

"How is everybody?" asked Jose with a smile on his boyish face.

"I feel lousy," said Annie, a large Jewish lady with hair dyed black. "I hate it when it rains. It makes me feel like killing myself."

"You don't really mean that, do you?" asked Jose. "Because if you do, I'll have to get somebody to call 911."

"No don't do that," snapped Annie. "I hate going to the hospital. They're like being in jail. And the bitch nurses are like wardens. They're probably all dykes any way."

"I have to be careful what I think," said Jason. "A scary thought can become reality."

Jason was a fairly recent newcomer to Campbell Care. He was a thin and tall young black man in his twenties. He did not seem to trust anyone very much. Paisley figured that he was a loner outside of the program.

"God bless America," said Kevin.

"You don't want to keep on going to the hospital, Annie," said Kenneth. "They'll send you to a permanent hospital like Overbook or Greystone. You should never say you want to kill yourself unless you really mean it."

"Why is everybody here criticizing me?" asked Annie. "I don't want to go back to that place like a jail."

"Have you ever been in jail, Annie?" asked Mark, a thirty-five-year-old Turkish man.

"No, not really," said Annie. "I couldn't stand being there unless my boyfriend could visit me."

"Then how do you know if the hospital is like a jail or not?" asked Mark.

"Stop criticizing me, Mark," said Annie who started to cry.

"Don't cry, Annie," said Jose assuredly. "He didn't mean to criticize you. He was just asking you a simple question."

"Okay, I'll stop crying," said Annie. "It's just that I've seen movies about jail, and they seem like Overbrook was."

Annie wiped away her tears with a white paper napkin that she had in her big, red purse. It matched the color of her lipstick.

"I know I was in Overbrook for eleven months," said Jason. "Then I was there again for another year."

"I was in Greystone for two years," said Jim. "My wife divorced me while I was there."

Jim had a pleasant baritone voice which Paisley liked very much. Paisley wondered if Jim could do voiceovers for movies and commercials.

"She is such a bitch," said Mark. "But then most women are bitches."

"You call women 'bitches,'" said Kevin. "You call men 'bastards.'"

"What do you mean?" said Annie. "I don't understand you."

"I don't even want to go there, dude," said Kenneth. "You said too much already."

"I don't think we should talk like that in here," said Jose. "You can talk about women in the men's group next time."

"Wars and plagues are from the devil," said Jason. "The devil sometimes hurts people who love God."

"In God we trust," said Kevin. "It even says it on the one-dollar bill in my pocket."

"Thank you, Kevin," said Jose.

Kevin and Lois both had a compulsive habit of saying things in groups that were not relevant to the topic being discussed. Jose and other staff members tried to say nice things to them.

"I don't like people who talk to me and then turn on me," said Annie. "That's two faced. I'm a good person."

"People are afraid of mentally ill patients because they are an unknown to them," said Jose. "You have to try to ignore the ignorant statements of mean people. That goes for every one of you in this room."

"God is on my side," said Jason. "He won't let anything bad happen to me."

"I noticed something the other day. Liza has a pierced tongue. Would you ever get your tongue pierced?" asked Paisley, looking at Jose.

"Are you asking me?" asked Jose. "No, I wouldn't but that's just my own personal preference."

"I don't see how anyone could get anything pierced besides their ears," said Mary. "It's weird. Liza is weird too. She better not touch me."

"And tattoos too," said Annie, "I think tattoos are okay on a man if he doesn't have too many. But tattoos on a woman are vulgar and unfeminine."

"I disagree with you on that one," said Gino. "A little rose on a woman's shoulder can be very sexy."

"I don't want to ever get a tattoo," said Kenneth. "I am part black and part Cherokee. So I am dark skinned."

"You can't get tattoos anyway," said Annie. "Your skin is so dark that they wouldn't show up."

"Maybe your right," said Kenneth. "I sometimes forget about that."

"Would you get your tongue pierced, Kenneth?" asked Mark.

"I consider that to be a very personal question," said Kenneth. "So, I'm not going to answer it."

"I wouldn't," said Jason. "But I do have a tattoo under my left eye."

Jason had a tattoo of a blue tear drop right under his left eye. Paisley heard that was sign that someone close to that man had died. It was similar to widows wearing black dresses for a year after their husbands died.

"I don't want any decorations on me. I'm not a Christmas tree, oh Christmas tree your branches are delightful," sang Kevin.

Several people laughed. Kevin never deliberately said anything that was funny. He also did not get upset when someone laughed at him.

"What do tattoos, and piercings have to do with social skills?" asked Jose.

"When you get the tattoos or piercings you have to talk to the tattooist about what kind of tattoo you want," said Jason "Also the needles have to be sterilized."

"You have to be assertive," said Paisley.

"You have to be crazy," said Annie.

"What kind of social skills are you all using right now in this group?" asked Jose.

"This is criticism," said Kenneth. "We know now that your looks can turn other people off. A tattoo can make you look cool to one person and ugly to another one."

"When you are waiting in line for breakfast or lunch you're using social skills," said Mary. "You're being patient and polite to the other people."

At that moment the door opened, and Polly stuck her head in saying, "Is Lucille Trimble in here? Her ICMS worker is here to see her."

"I think she's in Room 10," said Jose.

"Okay. Thank you," said Polly. "Have a nice day everyone!"

Polly closed the door.

"Was Polly using any social skills just now?" asked Jose after the door closed.

"Yes, she was," said Paisley. "She was following rules of etiquette, by saying 'Thank you' and 'Have a nice day!'"

"What is etiquette?" asked Mark, for whom English was a second language.

"It's about manners," said Mary. "Manners are something that many people in this place sorely lack."

"They're lacking and lackadaisical," said Kevin.

"In what other ways do you use social skills during the day?" asked Jose.

"When dealing with your noisy neighbors you are using social skills," said Paisley. "Before I moved to my own apartment, I told my Easter Seals case worker about the incident. She tells the landlady who then tells the neighbor that he needs to keep the noise level down."

"That's a very good example Paisley," said Jose.

"Back in the old days people were more concerned about etiquette," said Mary. "I know that from reading old novels like Charles Dickens when we were in high school."

"How is that different?" asked Jose. "His books are really old school."

"Some of the guys I knew were getting high in high school," said Kevin blithesomely.

"In the past women couldn't wear slacks like the ones that I'm wearing," said Mary. "They were only allowed to wear dresses."

"Only prostitutes and actresses wore make up," said Gino. "Now anyone can look like a slut."

"Woman didn't wear their hair short until the Roaring Twenties," said Paisley. "And until then it was considered unladylike for women to smoke cigarettes. Hollywood changed a lot of things for women, and we've never gone back since then."

"I hadn't thought of that before," said Jose.

"When a child died people would put a black wreath on their front door. And they would use stationary lined in black because they were in mourning," added Paisley.

"Oh dear, what can I do? Baby's in black and I'm feeling blue," said Kevin from an old Beatles song. "Tell me oh, what can I do?"

"Where does he get his stuff from?" asked Jose.

"Kevin's a little older than me," said Jim "And he remembers songs from back in the day. Like The Beatles, The Hollies, The Beau Brummels."

"Oh, I see," said Jose. "I was born in 1986."

"That was ten years after the Bicentennial celebration," said Mary. "That makes you 25 years old."

"I was living with my father in Manhattan," said Paisley. "He and I went to Hudson River to see all of the tall ships. It was really beautiful."

"I can imagine," said Mary. "I saw that on TV news."

"You're moved a lot, haven't you?" asked Jim.

"Yes, I have, Jim," replied Paisley "I've lived in New York, New Jersey, Maryland, Washington, D.C. and Connecticut."

"I've only lived in Japan, New Jersey, and South Carolina," said Jim.

"Are you moving down south soon?" asked Annie.

"Yes, I am," said Jim.

"Where are you going to move to?" asked Jose.

"I'm moving to Chamberlain, South Carolina," said Jim. "I'm going to live with my mother."

"Why are you moving?" asked Annie.

"My boarding home is being sold in a month," said Jim. "So, I thought it would be a good time to go back to my roots."

"We're all going to miss you," said Jose. "You're such a great guy."

"I'm going to miss you too," said Annie. "I don't want you to move."

"Are you crying?" asked Jose.

"Yes, I am," said Annie. "I need a hug."

Jim stood up and hugged Annie.

"I don't want to see you go either," intoned Kenneth. "But I know it is what you really want."

"I'll stay in touch," said Jim. "Maybe somebody can come down and visit me some day."

Jim released Annie who wiped away her tears. They both sat down again.

"I don't want you to leave too," said Mary who was also crying.

"Oh God," said Jason. "I feel so sad all of a sudden."

"A lot of people are going to miss you, Jim," said Jose. "A lot of people care about you."

"I'll miss you very much," said Annie, dabbing her eyes with a white paper napkin, "I love you like a brother. The brother from another mother?"

"I don't know what to say," said Jim calmly, "I never imagined that people would be so upset over my leaving."

"Does that mean you'll change your mind?" asked Paisley.

Jim took a moment to respond. Paisley felt his heart sink. Annie and Mary both started to cry tenderly.

"No Paisley," said Jim, gently patting Paisley's shoulder. "It's time for me to move on. That doesn't mean that we can't still be friends."

Paisley decided not to cry, although he felt that way.

"I'm glad we went to New York City before you left," said Paisley wistfully.

"Have we been using social skills today?" asked Jose.

"More than that," said Gino. "Annie and Mary have been using their crying skills. They are such wusses."

"Are you making fun of me?" snapped Annie.

"No, Annie," said Jose. "Nobody is making fun of anybody."

"God grant me the serenity to accept the things I cannot change," said Kevin, who was in the M.I.C.A. group. "Courage to change the things I can and wisdom to know the difference."

"Very good Kevin," said Jose. "You remembered the Serenity Prayer."

"My mother used to have that on her wall in the kitchen," said Paisley. "On top of the plaque with the quote was a pair of praying hands."

"I got sick when my mother died," said Annie. "I still miss her very much."

"Oh, please don't get her started again," said Mary. "I am so bored of her."

"Courage to accept the things that I cannot change," quoted Jose. "That's true for everybody, Annie, not just alcoholics. Everyone passes away some day."

"Jose's right," said Kenneth soothingly. "You and Mary need to accept things that you can't change like Jim's moving and your mother's dying."

"But it's so hard sometimes," said Annie.

"I know it is," said Kenneth "My father was murdered. Imagine how hard that was to get over that they never found the killer."

"That's terrible," said Jose.

"You're right, Jose," said Annie "I'm not the only one who's had a hard time. It's also hard being a diabetic."

"I know," said Paisley "I'm diabetic too, Annie. My mother and her father were also diabetic, and also had high blood pressure like me. At least I don't have to inject insulin every day like they did."

"I should hate to have to take insulin every day," said Annie.

"See, Annie in some ways you're lucky too," said Jose. "Your father wasn't murdered like Kenneth's, and you don't have to take insulin like Paisley's mother."

"Exactly," said Kenneth "You have some things to be thankful for."

"I understand it all now," agreed Annie.

"You've had it easy compared to me," said Mark. "I came here from Turkey when I was sixteen. I had an alcoholic father and had to learn to speak English. Don't be so whiny."

"Okay, I get the picture," said Annie coolly.

"Is everyone feeling all right now?" asked Jose.

"Yes, I think so," said Annie.

"I'm okay," said Mark.

The bell rang ending this period. Everyone left Room 2 except for Paisley, Kenneth, and Jim.

"I'm sorry if I put on the spot, Jim," said Paisley. "I have to get used to the idea that you have to leave."

"I want to be near to my brothers and sister," said Jim. "I almost never see them. And I also miss my mother. Since my father died, she gets lonely sometimes."

"I didn't realize that."

"I had no idea that people were so concerned over my leaving."

"A lot of people here like you and don't want you to go including me," said Kenneth.

"I appreciate that."

"Most of all I'd miss our pleasant trips to Manhattan."

"Yes, I will too."

"You promise that you'll stay in touch, Jim?"

"Yes, I will Paisley. I'll send you two my address and phone number when I get down south. Okay?"

"Okay, I care about you very much, Jim and I want you to say in my life forever."

"Thank you, Paisley. I'll always be your friend."

"When exactly are you moving?"

"In two weeks."

Chapter 19

Paisley endured the last two weeks before Jim's departure as stoically as possible. However, he felt as though it was raining in his heart like the poem by Paul Verlaine. He dreaded Jim's leaving not knowing when he would ever see him again. He had seen Jim every day at Campbell Care and soon he would no longer be there.

Jim possessed all the qualities that Paisley wanted in a man. He was intelligent and kind. He had a soothing voice which always appealed to him. He had a nice cafe au lait complexion. Soon all that Paisley would have would be the sound of his disembodied voice over the telephone wires. Or perhaps through emails online?

Going to his program would not be as appealing anymore. Although he still had friends at Campbell Care whom he liked very much, Paisley would miss Jim greatly. It just would not be the same experience anymore.

The thought that Jim would leave forever made Paisley feel a heaviness in his chest and a desire to cry. He thought in workshop this is the last time I'll even do flours with Jim. This is also going to be the last time that I'll eat lunch with him in the APR.

At lunch time, that last day they would be together, they ate meat loaf, mashed potatoes and corn. As they sat at one of the wooden tables with the foldable metal legs, Jim looked at Paisley.

"What are you thinking Paisley?"

"I don't want you to leave," said Paisley.

Just then Kenneth sat down in one of the eight seats around the table. The plastic chairs had chrome legs and a seat that was contoured to fit one's backside. They were easy to clean in case someone accidentally peed or threw up on them.

"I remember that you're leaving Campbell Care soon," said Kenneth putting ketchup on his meatloaf.

"Yes, I am," said Jim.

"Why don't you just transfer to another program?" asked Kenneth. "Campbell Care is not the only one in New Jersey. I heard of one called Northwest Essex Community Healthcare."

"No, Kenneth I'm not just going to another program," responded Jim. "I'm leaving New Jersey altogether."

"You are?" asked Kenneth.

"Yes, I am."

"Jim mentioned this plan to me before," said Paisley. "But I hoped that maybe Jim would change his mind and decide to stay in New Jersey at Campbell Care."

"Why are you leaving?" asked Kenneth taking a bite from his meat loaf.

"I want to be near to my brothers and sisters. I almost never see them being up here."

"Who are you going to live with?" asked Kenneth.

"My mother has a house down in South Carolina in a little town called Chamberlain."

"My great grandmother's maiden name was Chamberlain," said Paisley. "I wonder if that town was founded by distant relatives of mine. Maybe you could look that up for me on the Internet."

"You have a computer?" asked Kenneth.

"Yes, I do. It was a gift from my brothers."

"So maybe you really could look that up on the internet for Paisley."

"Yeah, I guess so."

Paisley took a sip from the 20-ounce diet coke which he brought ever morning to slake his thirst. Dry mouth was one of the symptoms of the psychiatric medications that he took every day for anxiety and depression. His heart was beginning to feel like a desert as well. He never realized himself how deeply he felt about Jim.

"I'm going to miss you and your diet sodas," said Jim.

"Paisley is definitely Mr. Soda Man," said Kenneth.

"I couldn't live without my soda," said Paisley. "I'd probably dry up into a little pile of dust without it."

They all laughed.

"Do you think that your mother would allow you to have visitors?" asked Paisley. "I've never been to South Carolina."

"It's really nice down there," explained Jim. "I'll have to ask my mother about that before I can give you a yes or no answer."

"I understand," said Paisley. "Since it's her home and not yours, you need to get her permission first. That makes a lot of sense to me."

"Don't worry about it, Paisley," added Jim consolingly. "I'm sure my mother will be okay with it, but I have to ask her first anyway. It's not like I'll be living with a roommate that I found through a personal ad or something."

"That's just part of etiquette," said Paisley. "To visit someone else's home, you need to see if they'll agree to having visitors or not."

"Does your mother know that Paisley is gay?" asked Kenneth.

At that moment an attractive Indian lady approached their table. It was Joy. Her kind personality made her name seem appropriate to everyone.

"I heard you're leaving us Jim," said Joy. "Is that true?"

"Yes, it is, Joy," said Jim. "I'm going to live with my mother in South Carolina."

"We're all going to miss you very much," said Joy. "Can't I go there with you?"

"I don't think so."

"I was only joking." Joy laughed. "I love you, Jim."

Joy bent over and kissed Jim on the left cheek.

"Thank you, Joy. I didn't know that you cared about me."

"Everyone loves you here, Jim," added Joy as she walked away. "Keep in touch. Don't be a stranger."

"I will."

Paisley had finished his lunch by now.

"Any way," said Kenneth. "Does your mother know Paisley is gay?"

"Yes," replied Jim. "But it isn't an issue with her anymore."

Jim took a bite of his meatloaf.

"So, you think she would let you have visitors?" asked Kenneth.

"Yes, I do," said Jim. "But I know that I should ask her first, especially if it's someone that she has never met before."

"Yeah, you don't want to just spring someone on her," said Paisley. "That would be disrespectful. It isn't because you know me through a mental health program, or is it?"

"Yes, it could be that," agreed Kenneth.

"I think my mother would like you Paisley," said Jim. "She likes whoever I like. She trusts me that way. That fact anyone I know has problems doesn't factor into the equation anymore."

"Okay," said Paisley.

"I promise I'll call both of you after I get down there and let you know what's up."

"Good. I'll look forward to your call."

"I'll have to talk to the director before I leave," explained Jim. "I need to get refills sent to the new pharmacy in South Carolina."

"Take care, Jim," said Kenneth.

"Thanks," replied Jim. "I will."

He got up and walked over to the assistant directors' office at the opposite end of the lunchroom. He knocked on the door and entered her office.

"I don't want to come here to Campbell Care after he leaves," said Paisley sadly. "Too many memories."

"I know what you, man," said Kenneth. "I am getting bored of this place any way."

Chapter 20

Paisley waited a week before he finally got what would turn out to be the most important call of his life. Kenneth asked him every day at Campbell Care whether Jim called yet about his visiting him in South Carolina. Each day of his waiting for a response seemed to pass with excruciating slowness. Would Paisley continue to live in New Jersey possibly forever as a confirmed bachelor? Or would the future hold the admittedly ambiguous possibility of companionship with a handsome and intelligent man whom Paisley truly loved? His fate was entirely dependent on Jim's decision to allow him to move down to South Carolina and stay with him.

Paisley had never lived down south before. He had lived in many places, more than he had ever anticipated before during his youth. He had lived in Connecticut, New York, Maryland, Virginia, Washington, D.C., and New Jersey. Despite his frequent moving, more than anyone else that he ever knew, Paisley truly despised moving. If he really did move to South Carolina to be with Jim, it would hopefully be the last time that he would ever move. Otherwise, Paisley would remain forever in New Jersey, because he now lived in a low-income apartment. He had found it through the Newark Housing Authority as all his friends had suggested.

Feeling bored, Paisley walked over from his comfortable single bed to the tall black dresser across the room. He turned on the radio to his favorite station WCBS FM 101.1. The song playing was *Some Day We'll be Together* by the Supremes. Paisley hoped that the song was an omen.

One day his creamy colored landline telephone finally rang. Paisley put the receiver up to his left ear, being right-handed.

"Hello. This is Paisley."

"Hi, Paisley. This is Jim."

"Yes, Jim."

"I have good news for you."

"Yes?"

"You can come to visit for as long as you want, Paisley."

"Do you really mean that?"

"Yes, I do," answered Jim cheerfully.

"I'll be there in a week. Is that okay with you?"

"Yes, that fine."

Paisley could feel his heart beating faster, realizing that his dream of living with Jim was really about to come true. It made him think of his favorite song by The Seekers called "I'll Never Find Another You."

"I need to give NHA some notice. Buy a one-way bus ticket. Pack my clothes etc. I think that I will mail my papers down separately."

"No problem."

"I'll see you soon, Jim."

"I'm looking forward to it."

"Me too. This will be my own forever after I guess."

"If that's what you want, Paisley then it might be. But you may have trouble adjusting to things down here."

"Yes, I know. I thought about that already. I'll see you in a week then."

"All right. Have a save trip down here."

"Thank you, Take care."

"You, too. Goodbye."

"Goodbye for the time being."

Paisley moved down to South Carolina to live with Jim and never had to move ever again. He had to endure a very long bus ride from New Jersey to South Carolina. It made several stops, including many places where he had lived before.

For example, the Greyhound bus stopped in Arlington, VA, Washington, D.C. Every few hours the driver would allow all the passengers to leave the bus at stops where there was a restaurant.

Paisley's family was glad that Paisley finally found what he was always looking for. Kenneth promised to visit eventually as well. Perhaps the three of them could find an apartment together in the future?